Quick & Easy EMF Guide

99 Tips

to Lower Exposure to
Harmful Electromagnetic Radiation

Includes Dangers of 5G & Smart Devices

LOIS CADWALLADER, MA

with **Bill** CADWALLADER, MBA, EMRS
Certified Electromagnetic Radiation Specialist

Stop Dirty Electricity
Las Vegas, Nevada

Quick & Easy EMF Guide
99 Tips to Lower Exposure to Harmful Electromagnetic Radiation,
Includes Dangers of 5G & Smart Devices

Copyright © 2020 by Lois Cadwallader

Stop Dirty Electricity
Las Vegas, Nevada
StopDirtyElectricity.com

ISBN-13: 978-1-7323650-5-6
ISBN-10: 1-7323650-5-9

Library of Congress Control Number: 2020909103

HEA021000: HEALTH & FITNESS / Safety

Printed in the United States of America

Disclaimer of Liability

Contents

Introduction

Electro-what?

Electromagnetic radiation is known by different names:

- Electro-smog
- Electro-pollution
- Electromagnetic Fields (EMFs)
- Electromagnetic Radiation (EMR)
- Dirty Electricity
- Electromagnetic Interference (EMI)
- Radio Frequency (RF)
- Wireless/WiFi/Bluetooth Radiation
- Microwave Radiation

Throughout this book, I will refer to all of the above as EMFs as I offer 99 useful tips to help you protect yourself and your family.

Although we cannot totally escape the presence of EMFs, we can take steps and adopt habits that will greatly reduce our exposure to harmful electromagnetic radiation. Most of the tips contained in this book are simple and free or nearly free. Most of these solutions can be implemented right away or in a very short time. They are scientific and measurable.

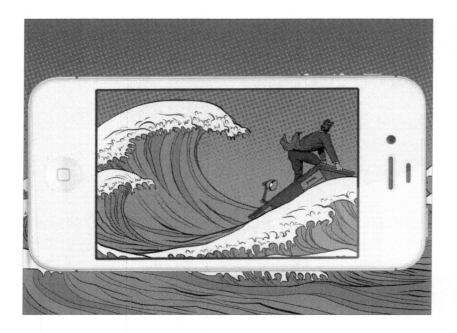

We all live in a sea of man-made electromagnetic radiation coming
- Through the AIR and
- From the WIRES.

How much is too much?
No one really knows for sure. But the fact is, there have been:
- No pre-market studies.
- No long-term studies.
- No opportunity for an individual to opt-out of this technology.
- It is EV-ery-where.

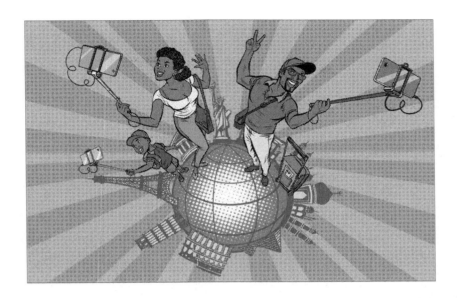

It has been demonstrated that all man-made EMFs, including ELFs (Extremely Low Frequencies) can:
- Break DNA single and double-strands
- Cause oxidative cell damage
- Disrupt cell metabolism and communication
- Break down the blood-brain barrier
- Reduce melatonin production
- Alter brain glucose metabolism
- Generate stress proteins
- Disrupt voltage-gated calcium channels

Just to name a few. And this is true for both wired and wireless EMFs.

All of the above health conditions are well-documented. (See Websites & Resources.) The debate is over whether or not the above effects on living cells *matter* to human health in a measurable way. And because people are not dropping dead right and left from using electronic technology, government and industry scientists contend that the above effects are not significant.

But the fact that all man-made EMFs do affect living cells should be a concern to us all, whether we are symptomatic or not. You probably bought this book because you already know, or at least suspect, that EMFs are harming us, our families, our environment, and even our pets. You are looking for things you can do right now that are quick, easy, and scientifically sound.

We have numerous assaults against our health, our immunity, our well-being. Let's not allow EMFs to possibly negatively tip the balance of our body's immune defense mechanisms.

As 5G is implemented, it will only make things worse, in that the smaller antennas can be brought very, very close to your home.

5G can include a type of microwave frequency called millimeter waves (MMW). These millimeter waves are the fastest, shortest, highest-intensity wave lengths within the microwave spectrum.

This is not just an upgrade of 4G. This is the next major evolution in wireless communication. 5G is the central platform for connecting everything to everyone at all times. It will be the necessary technological support for all things "smart."

Here are some of the crucial elements to implementing 5G:

- Density: Network density (i.e., adding more base stations and access points) will be necessary to get network access closer to individual users—along city streets, in buildings, and everywhere in between. That means adding more antennas and small cell sites. Cell towers can now be as close as 250 feet, or one every three to twelve homes in urban or suburban areas, mounted on lampposts. Speeds will be over 20 times faster than the current 4G technology.

- Virtualization: To effectively manage the spectrum, physical equipment will shift to virtualized environments operating in centralized data centers using solutions such as centralized radio access networks (C-RAN), network function virtualization (NFV), and cell virtualization.
- Aggregation: Carrier aggregation combines multiple component carriers across the available spectrum to combine chunks of bandwidth, increase data rates, and improve network performance.
- Massive Multiple Input/Multiple Output (MIMO): Thousands of active antenna elements will work together to provide MIMO.
- Your Smartphone as a Smart HUB: The super high-speed mobile broadband access and truly ubiquitous, laser-sharp coverage will let all of your smart devices communicate directly with one another and your 5G smartphone will act as the Hub. Think of your smartphone as the ultimate universal remote.
- Low Latency: No wait-time for video streaming. Very high reliability, global coverage.

In addition to bringing sources of electromagnetic radiation closer to us, it provides an avenue for extreme surveillance. 5G is one of the most insidious invasions of privacy ever promoted. Privacy will be lost, almost to the point of extinction. This is Big Brother on steroids.

This new technology, like previous iterations, remains untested and unavoidable. There is no "opt-out" program.

What's it doing to our health and how much radiation should we subject ourselves to?

Remember the novel coronavirus? The COVID-19 pandemic? Like EMFs, we couldn't see, touch, or smell that invisible enemy. Now is a good time to unburden and protect our immune system as much as possible.

These tips are best implemented in a single, free-standing dwelling. If you live in an apartment complex or attached living space, these remediation tips will be less effective due to radiation spill-over from your neighbors. But do what you can, because even small changes can reap great reductions in EMF levels.

If you want the entire backstory, the history of collusion and cover-up between industry and government, the research, and expanded solutions, check out the book I co-authored, *EXPOSED: The Electronic Sickening of America and How to Protect Yourself — Includes Dangers of 5G & Smart Devices.*

But if you just want to know the short story—what to do right now, this is the right book to read.

Let's get started.

—Lois Cadwallader
Las Vegas, Nevada

Zzzzzz – Protect Your Sleeping Area

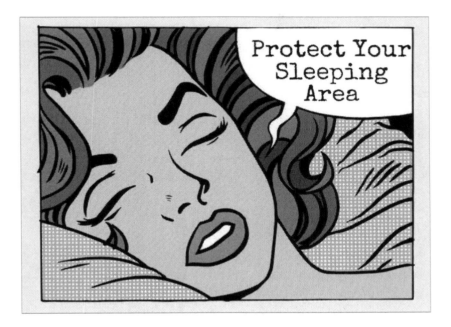

1 Move your cell-phone charging stations out of the bedrooms or as far away as possible. This is #1 for a reason. Most people do not realize that they are being exposed to radiation from the charging cords as well as wireless radiation from their cell phones. A cell phone emanates dangerous levels of radiation 24/7 even when not in use.

2 Move your router as far away as possible from sleeping and living areas.

3 Turn off your router / WiFi at night. You can use a timer or remote-control outlet switch to make this easy. Cost? Less than $9.00.

4 Or, better yet, turn your router and WiFi on *only* when you need it.

5 Make your sleeping area as "low-tech" as you can. Kill the power to all electronics at night. This would include TVs, speakers, etc. (See Comprehensive Home Safety Audit – Bedroom.) Again, you can use a timer or remote-control outlet switch to make this easy.

6 Unplug lamps, clocks, etc., that are near your sleeping area. Again, you can use a timer or remote-control outlet switch for ease of use.

7 If you really want to get serious, turn off circuit breakers during sleeping hours. (Make sure critical devices such as an alarm system, medical devices, and refrigerator are not affected.)

8 Use a "sleeping canopy," which works well and is kind of cool looking. But it costs some money. You can find a sleeping canopy online at www.slt.co. (Use code safe7 for 5% off.)

9 Limit screen time before you go to sleep. The blue light emanating from the screen, in addition to the EMFs, interrupts sleep and decreases melatonin production. You can also purchase blue-light-blocking glasses and screen covers.

10 Remove electric blankets and electric sleeping pads from your bed. Be sure to completely unplug them.

11 Replace beds with metal inner springs with non-metal materials.

12 If you have an electric bed, unplug it when you sleep. Or, as mentioned above, use a remote-control outlet switch to turn off the power to the bed when you sleep.

Note: Tip #78—use dirty electricity plug-in filters—is particularly important to apply to your sleeping area. I list it under Advanced Solutions because the filters do need to be ordered and cost $29 per filter. But it is something you can do immediately to reduce radiation from dirty electricity.

NOTES

Distance Is Your Friend

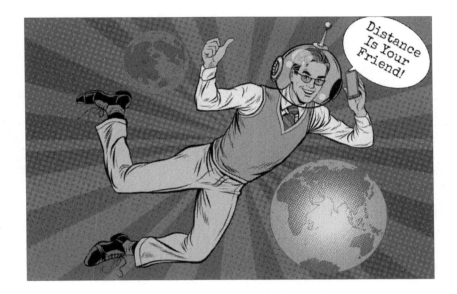

13 When talking on a cell phone or other electronic communication device, use speaker-phone mode whenever possible. I understand that this is not possible if you are in a noisy place, but try not to put your cell phone next to your ear.

14 When possible, locate cell phones or tablets as far away as possible from your body when not in use.

15 Move your chair away from the wall when sitting. Unseen wiring in your wall could be a source of EMFs.

16 Check the wall in back of your bed. If there is a breaker box, utility meter, or air conditioning / heating unit on or near the wall where you place your head on the pillow, rearrange your bed so that it is away from those things. If possible, move 6-8 feet away from those items, as they can produce high levels of magnetic radiation.

17 Move your pet's bed away from the wall. If possible, move it 6-8 feet away from a wall. And make sure your pet's bed is away from all wireless devices.

18 If you must use a microwave oven, leave the room when it is on. And don't forget your pets. How far? Go to: www.StopDirtyElectricity.com and scroll down to the bottom to view a 1-minute video.

19 If you use a medical device, move it as far away from your body as the cord will allow.

20 Distance is your friend. Whenever possible, increase distance from all electronics, both wired and wireless devices.

21 Place your work station/computer on a rolling desk or casters, and roll it away from the wall and electrical cords when using.

22 Avoid living or working close to high-voltage power lines. Try to be at least ¼ mile away. This should be measured. (See Websites & Resources.)

23 Avoid living or working close to a cell tower. Try to be at least one mile away. This should be measured. See Antenna Search: http://www.antennasearch.com for cell towers within two miles.

NOTES

Practice Safe Tech

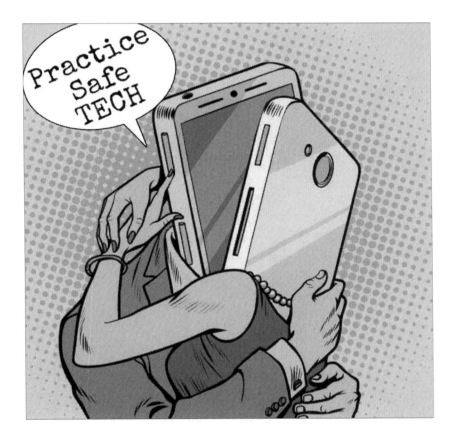

24 When carrying your cell phone on your body, turn Airplane Mode ON and Bluetooth and WiFi OFF. This is the only safe way to carry a cell phone. (Note—you will not receive phone calls, text messages, or data in this mode, so remember to reverse this when you are no longer carrying your phone on your body.)

25 Important—many new devices have an auto-reconnect, so you must check periodically to ensure that Airplane Mode remains ON and Bluetooth and WiFi remain OFF.

26 Download books, music, videos, and games. Enjoy with Airplane Mode ON and Bluetooth and WiFi OFF.

27 Don't entrust your safety to a "shielding case." Think about it—if you are able to make or receive a call, the radiation has to leak out somewhere. And your phone normally has to work harder to get a signal with a case on. A shielding case could actually intensify the radiation. Some shielding cases are better than others. If you choose to use one, it should be measured.

28 Avoid using portable electronic devices on your lap. Instead, place on a table as far away as possible. You can even hard wire your portable devices to an Ethernet connection.

29 Use electronics in battery mode and not plugged in. Remember, EMFs come from WIRES as well as through the AIR. Batteries are usually not a problem.

Go Retro

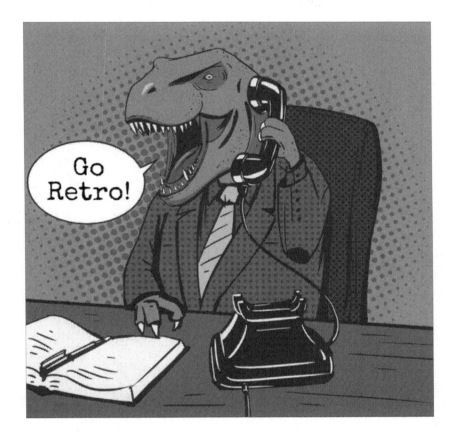

30 Replace fluorescent, CFL, and LED lighting with incandescent or incandescent halogen light bulbs. Make sure that the halogen light bulbs are the kind with the wide screw-in base.

31 If you have dimmer switches, turn them completely OFF when not using, not just "down." And if you are not "married" to your mood lighting, replace them with a regular on/off switch.

32 Maintain a landline phone if possible. You can forward your cell phone calls to your landline.

33 Replace all cordless phones with corded landline phones. Make sure there is no cordless handset. The cordless phone base emanates dangerous levels of radiation 24/7, even when not in use.

34 Reject the "Smart Home" concept. Maintain older appliances that do not have wireless sensors; i.e., no "smart" appliances.

35 If you must purchase a new appliance, research a new but older model that does not have wireless sensors ... while they can still be found.

36 Get wired—hard wire electronic devices whenever possible instead of relying on wireless technology.

37 Replace a wireless mouse with a wired mouse.

38 Replace a wireless keyboard with a wired keyboard.

39 Hard wire your printer. You still need to disable the wireless sensor embedded in a printer. This is difficult but doable. Check the owner's manual or call the manufacturer.

40 Or, if it's easier, just cut the power at the outlet to your printer when not in use. You can purchase a remote-control outlet switch. Cost? Less than $9.00.

41 Use Ethernet cable instead of WiFi/wireless. There are Ethernet adapters for most portable electronic devices.

42 Resist "smart speakers," Bluetooth speakers, and other "Smart Home" gadgets. These things are pervasive and you may not be aware of how many things might be "smart." (See Comprehensive Home Safety Audit.)

NOTES

Just Say No

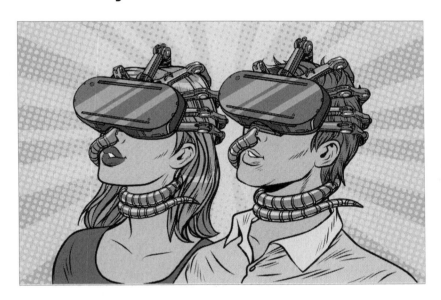

43 Just say NO to the 5G phone "upgrade."

44 Do not wear a wireless fitness device/smart watch. If you must wear one, at least take it off at night or when you are not exercising.

45 Never use a Bluetooth wireless ear piece. If you must use one, turn off and remove it from your ear immediately when you are not using it. Use a wired earpiece instead.

46 Never use wireless headphones. If you must use them, turn them off and immediately remove them from your head when not using them. Use a wired headphone set instead.

47 Attention, "gamers"—never use Virtual Reality or Augmented Reality wireless headsets. Use wired ones.

48 "Gamers" should use wired controls. Make sure you disable the wireless feature.

49 Try not to use electronic devices in a moving car, train, or subway. Wait till you depart the transportation vehicle to use device or check messages.

50 If you are electromagnetic hypersensitive and you must use the GPS feature on your phone while traveling, type in the address, then turn Airplane Mode ON and Bluetooth and WiFi OFF. This gives you most of the features of your GPS.

51 If you have an electrical utility "smart meter" with a digital display, tell your utility company you want to "opt out" and return to an analog meter. (There is a fee, which varies from state to state.)

Are You EMF Sensitive?

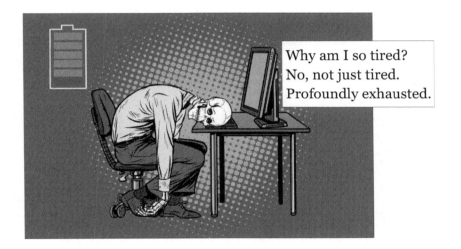

> Why am I so tired?
> No, not just tired.
> Profoundly exhausted.

Do You Have EHS? (Electromagnetic Hypersensitivity)

EMFs affect all of us at a cellular level, whether or not we are symptomatic. But some people are highly sensitive to electromagnetic radiation. It's as if they are allergic to EMFs.

Take note of the following:

✓ Do I live with a malaise of undiagnosed, vague symptoms? (headaches, nausea, dizziness, heart palpitations, weakness, "buzzing" feeling, to name just a few.)

✓ Do I notice a difference in my symptoms after use of technology?

✓ Have I ruled out other possible medical conditions with a health professional?

✓ Why am I worse in certain rooms or locations?
✓ Is there a place where my symptoms are particularly worse?
✓ Do I feel better when I am away from my home?
✓ Is there a place where my symptoms recede or disappear altogether?
✓ Do my symptoms go away when I am visiting other locations?

52 Pursue excellent nutritional support.

53 Limit the time that you use any type of electronic device as much as possible. Turn Airplane mode ON and Bluetooth and WiFi OFF.

54 Distance yourself from all electronics as much as possible.

55 Consult an EMF-aware health professional.

56 Consider shielded clothing if you are extremely sensitive to EMFs.

57 Consider adjusting your sleeping area to a less EMF-dense location.

58 Hire a Certified Electromagnetic Radiation Specialist as a consultant. If you are EHS, seek help early. You have some time before the 5G infrastructure is fully established and activated. It will only get worse as 5G is fully implemented.

59 One of the world's leading experts on EHS is Lloyd Burrell. Check out his website: www.Electricsense.com.

60 Avoid Unproven EMF remediation gadgets. As a long-time telemarketing friend once admitted, "Good for selling; not for buying."

Pendants, oils, decals, and dots may lull you into a fall sense of safety. The only proven way to reduce or eliminate harm from EMFs is to reduce or eliminate exposure levels, both through the AIR and from the WIRES.

OK, if you like those things, and you feel better wearing them, go ahead. Just don't make "subtle energy devices" your *sole* method of defense. You still need to bring down your level of EMF exposure. And that's scientific and measurable.

To check their benefits after reducing as much EMFs as possible, use them for 1-2 weeks and see how you feel. Then don't use them for 1-2 weeks and see how you feel.

NOTES

Unplug

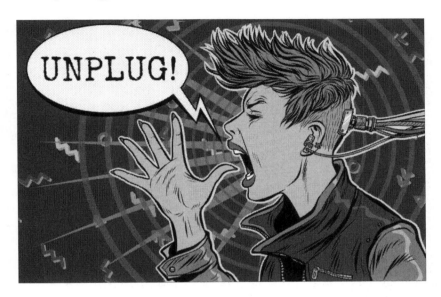

61 Cut the power to electronics and appliances whenever you are not using them. (Remember, EMFs come from electrical cords and cables as well as from WiFi, wireless, and Bluetooth, *even when they are not in use.*)

You can use a power strip and cut the power to appliances when not in use. Or, you can use a remote-control outlet switch. Or, simply unplug things that you are not using.

62 If you have an electric recliner, you can adjust it to a comfortable position. You can use a remote-control outlet switch to then cut the power and you can sit safely in your electric recliner. Just switch the power back on to re-adjust the position. Cost? Less than $9.00.

63 Take a "tech day off." Disconnect from all electronic devices, both wired and wireless as much as possible. Practice this on a regular basis. (This is an interesting concept called 24/6: Take a tech day off once a week. https://www.24sixlife.com/resources)

64 Look for opportunities to take advantage of natural sunlight when possible.

65 Spend as much time as possible outdoors in a natural environment.

Protecting Our Children

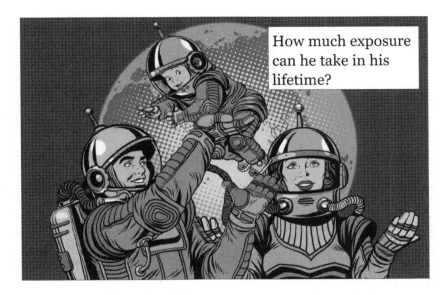

How much exposure can he take in his lifetime?

66 I recommend that you do not use a wireless baby monitor. If you use one, it must be measured to determine whether there is a safe distance for both the baby and the parent. Check out this 1-minute video to see the radiation danger of a wireless baby monitor: https://youtu.be/aH-fOn_i5dM

See Tech Wellness for a low-EMF baby monitor: https://techwellness.com/ (Use code safe7 for 5% off.)

67 Resist the high-tech baby stuff, like WiFi diapers, Bluetooth baby bottles, wireless pacifiers, etc., and just keep things simple. (See a list of possible wireless baby devices under Nursery in the Comprehensive Home Safety Audit Section.)

68 Ramp up physical touch, hugs, and conversations with intentional eye contact.

Read my article, "How Modern Technology Is Destroying Our Children's Health And What To Do About It," at: https://www.electricsense.com/technology-destroying-health/

69 Do not allow young children unlimited access to electronics of any kind, wired or wireless.

70 Remove all electronics from the dinner table and the bedrooms.

71 Let your older children know that this is important to you and to their safety and health—and that you are not eliminating technology, but helping them learn to master it.

72 Involve your children in deciding which steps they will take to lower radiation exposure and gain control over electronic device intrusion. Baby steps, baby steps. You could even tie in their "allowance" to checking off tips in this book.

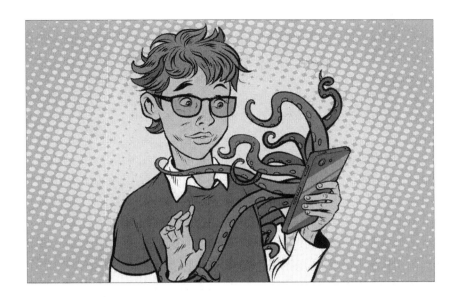

73 Let your teens research and explore high-interest issues such as surveillance, 5G controversies, the rise of GBM brain tumors, reproductive damage from EMF exposure, environmental damage, etc. Get edgy about this. (See Websites & Resources.) And check out my article, "Is Your Cell Phone Spying on You" at: https://www.electricsense.com/cell-phone-spying/

74 Get input from your children and agree on more low-tech family fun—hiking, biking, cooking, board games, concerts, travel, sports, etc.

75 Suggest to your teens that *not* being available via electronics 24/7 might be a "cool" thing, adding a certain "mystique" or "independence" to their social media persona.

76 If you suspect serious digital addiction, you may want to seek professional help.

77 Read, read, read to your young children.

Advanced Solutions

Most of the previous tips are things you can do on your own and require very little time and money. This section contains *very important* steps in decreasing your exposure to EMFs. But these actions require a higher level of commitment—when you are ready.

78 Use dirty electricity plug-in filters to lower EMFs in areas where you sleep, stand, or sit for any length of time. They are very effective. Of all the actions in this section, I would recommend dirty electricity plug-in filters as your first purchase.

However, three bits of caution:

1. Dirty electricity filters effectively lower dirty electricity. But on occasion they can raise magnetic fields, if wiring errors exist. If this happens, consult a Certified Electromagnetic Radiation Specialist for remediation.

2. There are some electromagnetic hypersensitive people who react better with one filter or the other. If you are EHS, you may want to compare how you feel with both filters and determine which one works best for you. Test them out. If you have a

negative reaction, pull them out and try the other type of filter. If neither is right for you, there are other filter options for some EHS people, but they are more expensive. Greenwave has a different type of filter that some EHS people seem to do better with, at the same price.

3. It rarely happens, but if you do feel worse when you plug in dirty electricity filters, remove them and call either a Certified Electromagnetic Radiation Specialist or the manufacturer of the filter for remediation.

So, even after the above cautions, I *do* use dirty electricity filters and they dramatically lower the dirty electricity from the wires. This is instantaneously and dramatically measurable.

There are two that I recommend:

✓ Greenwave dirty electricity filters, which can be purchased at: www.greenwavefilters.com (Use code safe7 for 5% off.)

✓ Stetzer dirty electricity filters, which can be purchased at: www.lessemf.com

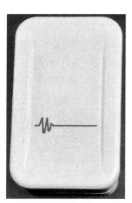

Stetzer filter

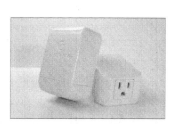

Greenwave filter

79

Measure—get good-quality EMF meters.

There are many reputable meters available. I recommend the ones below because they are good quality, easy to acquire, simple to use, and affordable.

Three meters will enable you to measure EMFs through the AIR and from the WIRES:

1. Radiation traveling through the AIR - WiFi, Wireless, Bluetooth, Smart Devices can be measured with either:

   ✓ Safe and Sound Classic

   OR

   ✓ Acousticom 2

Both of these meters can be purchased at: www.slt.co (Use code safe7 for 5% off.)

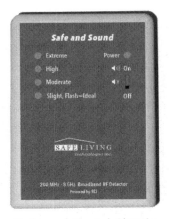

Safe and Sound Classic meter

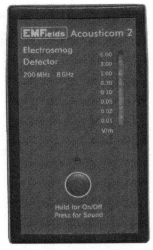

Acousticon 2 meter

2. Radiation from the WIRES—Electric Radiation and Magnetic Radiation can both be measured by:

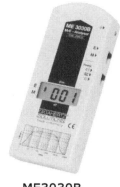

ME3030B
meter

  ✓ ME3030B
    It can be purchased at:
    www.slt.co (Use code safe7 for 5% off.)

3. Also from the WIRES—Dirty Electricity can be measured by either

  ✓ Greenwave EMI Meter
    It can be purchased at:
    www.greenwavefilters.com
    (Use code safe7 for 5% off.)

    OR

  ✓ Stetzer Meter
    It can be purchased at: www.lessemf.com

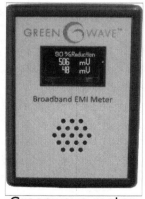

Greenwave meter

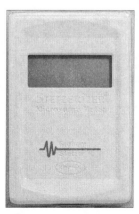

Stetzer meter

These three meters will give you measurements for all types of EMFs, both through the AIR and from the WIRES. There are many resources available to help you correctly use the meters, determine what are the safer levels to strive for, and how to do advanced remediation. You can do this. *EXPOSED: The Electronic Sickening of America and How to Protect Yourself – Includes Dangers of 5G & Smart Devices* includes more details on how to use meters as well as the optimal safety ranges for each type of EMF. More information at: www.StopDirtyElectricity.com

80 Consider shielding if you are in a high-EMF zone (near a cell tower, 5G antenna, near a business or neighbor with inescapable pollution of routers, smart devices, etc.) Shielding options include: Fabric, paint, window film, foil. These items can be purchased at: www.slt.co (Use code safe7 for 5% off.)

81 It is very important to contact a Certified Electro-magnetic Radiation Specialist for consultation, especially if you want to pursue shielding, as this can get tricky. Plan your shielding materials with the help of a qualified EMF professional. Find an Expert through the Building Biology Institute: https://buildingbiologyinstitute.org/find-an-expert/

82 Wrap your router with shielding fabric. You can measure to find out how many "wraps" it will take to reduce the EMFs coming from your router yet maintain functionality. Or, you can use your wireless device and keep wrapping until you don't have a signal. Then just unwrap until you get the signal strength necessary to use the device. Sources for advanced products are:

- ✓ Safe Living Technologies at: www.slt.co (Use code safe7 for 5% off.)
- ✓ Less EMF at: www.tinyurl.com/ExposedLessEMF
- ✓ Tech Wellness features low EMF products, such as a baby monitor, faraday bag, etc. https://techwellness.com/ (Use code safe7 for 5% off.)

83 Schedule a home inspection/remediation visit. Find an Expert through the Building Biology Institute: https://buildingbiologyinstitute.org/find-an-expert/

When my husband does a home inspection, he offers good, better, and best solutions that are scientific and measurable.

Comprehensive Home Safety Audit

Identifying Potential Sources of Radiation Through the Air and From the Wires

C all me crazy, but I think this is the most compre-hensive EMF checklist in existence. I wanted to be sure that no EMFs go undetected. My husband keeps up on every cutting-edge innovation that could possibly show up in your home. He attends the Consumer Electronics Show every year in Las Vegas, as well as the largest cell-phone conference in the United States, the Mobile World Congress in Southern California.

One of the speakers at a Mobile World Congress proudly announced that he found more than 60 "smart" devices in his home, and that was just walking around looking. These lists will help you begin to systematically rout out all the unknown, unthought-of electronics that are invisibly polluting your living area.

Remember: **A little + a little + a little = a LOT**

This list is exhaustive. And it could be exhausting. Just take it one room at a time so you don't get overwhelmed. Prioritize the order in which you go depending on where you spend most of your time . . . or whether you have children. Most people start with the bedroom, as protecting your sleep is of utmost importance.

Take a thorough inventory of both wireless and wired electronics, room-by-room, and decide what steps you can take today.

84

Bedroom: Radiation through the AIR—WiFi/Wireless/ Bluetooth/Smart Devices

Some of the below devices can have a WiFi, Wireless, Bluetooth, or Smart component in them. Normally, there is an interaction with a Smartphone.

☐ Air Filters – Smart
☐ Air Purifier
☐ Alarm Clock sound & vibration
☐ Anti-Snoring Device – Smart
☐ Bed Pad – Smart
☐ Bed Speakers
☐ Bedwetting Alarm
☐ Blu-ray DVD Player
☐ Cable Box
☐ Camera
☐ Ceiling Fan
☐ Ceiling Lamp with Speaker
☐ Ceiling Light Fixture
☐ Cell Phone
☐ Charger – Wireless

☐ Chargers
☐ Clock
☐ Control Buttons – Smart
☐ Cordless Phone
☐ CPAP Machines
☐ Digital Media Player
☐ Dimmer Switches
☐ Door Locks
☐ DVR
☐ Earbuds
☐ eBook Readers
☐ EKG Patch
☐ Essential Oil Diffuser
☐ Fan – Portable
☐ Fertility Tracker
☐ Fetal Monitor
☐ Fetus Camera
☐ Fetus Monitoring Band

☐ Fragrance Disseminator
☐ Gaming Systems
☐ Glasses – Smart
☐ HDTV Transmitter
☐ Headband Headset
☐ Head Phones – Wireless
☐ Heater – Portable
☐ Home Air Quality Monitor
☐ Home Audio
☐ Home Automation Item Tracker
☐ Home Devices – Smart
☐ Home Hub for all devices
☐ Home Sensing Carpet
☐ Intercom
☐ Internet Streaming Device
☐ Internet TV Device
☐ Internet Video Service
☐ iPad/Tablet/Kindle
☐ Lamps – Smart
☐ Laptop
☐ Light Bulb and Speaker
☐ Light Bulbs – Smart
☐ Light Switch
☐ Lighting Systems
☐ Mattress Cover – Smart
☐ Media Streamers
☐ Meditation Tracker
☐ Medical Monitoring

☐ Motion Detector
☐ Motorized Window Blinds
☐ MP3 Player
☐ Open or Close Door or Window Sensor
☐ Pillow for Snoring – Smart
☐ Plug Adaptor/Controller
☐ Power Strip – Smart
☐ Projector
☐ Remote Door Bell Chime
☐ Remote Thermostat Sensors
☐ Robot Vacuum
☐ Satellite Receiver
☐ Sauna
☐ Security Camera
☐ Security Lighting
☐ Security – Virtual Roommate
☐ Senior Home Health Monitoring
☐ Signal Booster/Extender
☐ Sleep Huggable Pillow
☐ Sleep monitoring System
☐ Sleeping Earphones
☐ Speakers – Smart
☐ Speakers – Wireless
☐ Thermostat – Smart
☐ TV

☐ TV Services
☐ Video Game Console

☐ Visual Enhancement
  Glasses
☐ Watch – Smart

Bedroom – Radiation from Wires – Electric Radiation, Magnetic Radiation & Dirty Electricity

☐ Plugged in Bluetooth
  Devices
☐ Plugged in WiFi Devices
☐ Plugged in Wireless
  Devices
☐ Plugged in Smart
  Devices

☐ Air Purifier
☐ Alarm Clock sound &
  vibration
☐ Bed Pad
☐ Bed Speakers
☐ Bedwetting Alarm
☐ Blu-ray DVD Player
☐ Cable Box
☐ Ceiling Fan
☐ Ceiling Lamp with
  Speaker
☐ Ceiling Light Fixture
☐ Charger - Wireless
☐ Chargers
☐ Clock
☐ Cordless Phone

☐ CPAP Machines
☐ Digital Media Player
☐ Dimmer Switches
☐ DVR
☐ Earbuds
☐ Electric Bed
☐ Electric Blanket
☐ Essential Oil Diffuser
☐ Extension Cords
☐ Fan – Portable
☐ Fragrance Disseminator
☐ Gaming Systems
☐ HDTV Transmitter
☐ Heater – Portable
☐ Heating Pad
☐ Home Air Quality
  Monitor
☐ Home Audio
☐ Home Automation Item
  Tracker
☐ Home Devices – Smart
☐ Home Hub for all
  devices
☐ Home Sensing Carpet

☐ Intercom
☐ Internet Streaming Device
☐ Internet TV Device
☐ Internet Video Service
☐ Lamps
☐ Light Bulb and Speaker
☐ Light Bulbs – Compact Fluorescent Lights (CFLs)
☐ Light Bulbs – Halogens – Small Base
☐ Light Bulbs – LEDs some
☐ Light Switch
☐ Lighting Systems
☐ Mattress Cover
☐ Media Streamers
☐ Meditation Tracker
☐ Medical Monitoring
☐ Motion Detector
☐ Motorized Window Blinds
☐ Plug Adaptor/Controller

☐ Power Strips
☐ Projector
☐ Remote Door Bell Chime
☐ Remote Thermostat Sensors
☐ Satellite Receiver
☐ Sauna
☐ Security – Virtual Roommate
☐ Security Camera
☐ Security Lighting
☐ Senior Home Health Monitoring
☐ Signal Booster/Extender
☐ Sleep Huggable Pillow
☐ Sleep monitoring System
☐ Sleeping Earphones
☐ Speakers
☐ Speakers – Smart
☐ Thermostat
☐ TV
☐ TV Services
☐ Video Game Console

85

Family Room/Living Room — WiFi/Wireless/ Bluetooth/Smart Devices

Some of the below devices can have a WiFi, Wireless, Bluetooth or Smart component in them. Normally there is an interaction with a Smartphone.

☐ Air Filters — Smart
☐ Air Purifier
☐ Blu-ray DVD Player
☐ Cable Box
☐ Ceiling Fan
☐ Ceiling Lamp with Speaker
☐ Ceiling Light Fixture
☐ Cell Phone
☐ Charger — Wireless
☐ Chargers
☐ Clock
☐ Cordless Phone
☐ Delivery Door — Smart
☐ Digital Media Player
☐ Dimmer Switches
☐ Door Locks
☐ DVR
☐ Earbuds
☐ eBook Readers
☐ Essential Oil Diffuser
☐ Fan — Portable
☐ Fragrance Disseminator
☐ Gaming Systems

☐ Glasses — Smart
☐ HDTV Transmitter
☐ Head Phones — Wireless
☐ Headband Headset
☐ Heater — Portable
☐ Home Air Quality Monitor
☐ Home Audio
☐ Home Automation Item Tracker
☐ Home Devices — Smart
☐ Home Sensing Carpet
☐ Humidifier — Portable
☐ Intercom
☐ Internet Streaming Device
☐ Internet TV Device
☐ Internet Video Service
☐ iPad/Tablet/Kindle
☐ Lamps — Smart
☐ Laptop
☐ Light Bulb and Speaker
☐ Light Bulbs — Smart
☐ Light Switch

☐ Lighting
☐ Lighting Systems
☐ Media Streamers
☐ Meditation Tracker
☐ Motion Detector
☐ Motorized Window Blinds
☐ MP3 Player
☐ Open or Closed Door or Window Sensor
☐ Plug Adaptor/Controller
☐ Projector
☐ Remote Door Bell Chime
☐ Remote Thermostat Sensors
☐ Robot Vacuum
☐ Satellite Receiver

☐ Sauna
☐ Security Camera
☐ Security Lighting
☐ Senior Home Health Monitoring
☐ Signal Booster/Extender
☐ Speakers – Smart
☐ Speakers – Wireless
☐ Standalone Streaming Services
☐ Thermostat – Smart
☐ TV
☐ TV Services
☐ Video Game Console
☐ Visual Enhancement Glasses
☐ Watch – Smart

Family Room/Living Room – Radiation from Wires – Electric Radiation, Magnetic Radiation & Dirty Electricity

☐ Plugged in Bluetooth Devices
☐ Plugged in WiFi Devices
☐ Plugged in Wireless Devices
☐ Plugged in Smart Devices

☐ Air Purifier
☐ Blu-ray DVD Player

☐ Cable Box
☐ Ceiling Fan
☐ Ceiling Lamp with Speaker
☐ Ceiling Light Fixture
☐ Ceiling Lights
☐ Charger – Wireless
☐ Chargers
☐ Clock
☐ Cordless Phone

- [ ] Digital Media Player
- [ ] Dimmer Switches
- [ ] DVR
- [ ] Essential Oil Diffuser
- [ ] Extension Cords
- [ ] Fan – Portable
- [ ] Fragrance Disseminator
- [ ] Gaming Systems
- [ ] HDTV Transmitter
- [ ] Heater – Portable
- [ ] Home Air Quality Monitor
- [ ] Home Audio
- [ ] Home Devices – Smart
- [ ] Home Hub for all devices
- [ ] Home Sensing Carpet
- [ ] Humidifier – Portable
- [ ] Internet Streaming Device
- [ ] Internet TV Device
- [ ] Internet Video Service
- [ ] Lamps
- [ ] Light Bulb and Speaker
- [ ] Light Bulbs – Compact Fluorescent Lights (CFLs)
- [ ] Light Bulbs – Halogens – Small Base
- [ ] Light Bulbs – LEDs some

- [ ] Light Switch
- [ ] Lighting
- [ ] Lighting Systems
- [ ] Media Streamers
- [ ] Meditation Tracker
- [ ] Motion Detector
- [ ] Motorized Window Blinds
- [ ] MP3 Player
- [ ] Plug Adaptor/Controller
- [ ] Power Strips
- [ ] Projector
- [ ] Remote Door Bell Chime
- [ ] Remote Thermostat Sensors
- [ ] Satellite Receiver
- [ ] Sauna
- [ ] Security – Virtual Roommate
- [ ] Security Camera
- [ ] Security Lighting
- [ ] Senior Home Health Monitoring
- [ ] Signal Booster/Extender
- [ ] Speakers
- [ ] Speakers – Smart
- [ ] Standalone Streaming Services
- [ ] TV
- [ ] TV Services
- [ ] Video Game Console

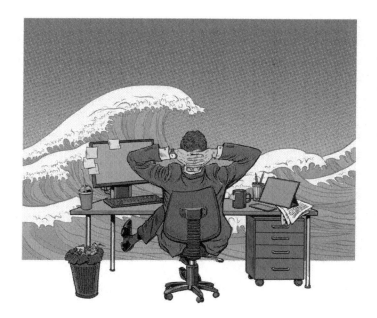

86

Home Office – WiFi/Wireless/Bluetooth/Smart Devices

Some of the below devices can have a WiFi, Wireless, Bluetooth or Smart component in them. Normally there is an interaction with a Smartphone.

☐ Air Filters – Smart
☐ Air Purifier
☐ Blu-ray DVD Player
☐ Cable Box
☐ Ceiling Fan
☐ Ceiling Lamp with
    Speaker
☐ Ceiling Light Fixture

☐ Cell Phone
☐ Charger – Wireless
☐ Chargers
☐ Clock
☐ Cloud Reusable
    Notebook
☐ Cordless Phone
☐ Digital Media Player

- ☐ Digitizer Pen
- ☐ Dimmer Switches
- ☐ Door Locks
- ☐ DVR
- ☐ Earbuds
- ☐ Ear Piece
- ☐ eBook Readers
- ☐ Essential Oil Diffuser
- ☐ Fan – Portable
- ☐ Fax Machine
- ☐ Fitness Chair
- ☐ Fragrance Disseminator
- ☐ Gaming Systems
- ☐ Glasses – Smart
- ☐ HDTV Transmitter
- ☐ Head Phones
- ☐ Headband Headset
- ☐ Headset
- ☐ Heater – Portable
- ☐ Home Air Quality Monitor
- ☐ Home Audio
- ☐ Home Automation Item Tracker
- ☐ Home Devices – Smart
- ☐ Home Hub for all devices
- ☐ Home Sensing Carpet
- ☐ Humidifier – Portable
- ☐ Intercom
- ☐ Internet Streaming Device
- ☐ Internet TV Device
- ☐ Internet Video Service
- ☐ iPad/Tablet/Kindle
- ☐ Keyboard - Wireless
- ☐ Label Maker
- ☐ Lamps – Smart
- ☐ Laptop
- ☐ Light Bulb and Speaker
- ☐ Light Bulbs – Smart
- ☐ Light Switch
- ☐ Lighting Systems
- ☐ Media Streamers
- ☐ Meditation Tracker
- ☐ Modem
- ☐ Motion Detector
- ☐ Motorized Window Blinds
- ☐ Mouse – Wireless
- ☐ MP3 Player
- ☐ Neckloops
- ☐ Open or Close Door or Window Sensor
- ☐ PC Tower
- ☐ Plug Adaptor/Controller
- ☐ Power Strip – Smart
- ☐ Printer
- ☐ Printer – 3D
- ☐ Projector
- ☐ Remote Door Bell Chime
- ☐ Remote Thermostat Sensors
- ☐ Robot Vacuum
- ☐ Router
- ☐ Satellite Receiver

☐ Sauna
☐ Security – Virtual
  Roommate
☐ Security Camera
☐ Security Lighting
☐ Senior Home Health
  Monitoring
☐ Signal Booster/Extender
☐ Speakers – Wireless
☐ Speakers – Smart
☐ Standalone Streaming
  Services

☐ Telephone Headset -
  Wireless
☐ Thermostat – Smart
☐ TV
☐ TV Services
☐ Video Game Console
☐ Visual Enhancement
  Glasses
☐ Watch – Smart
☐ Wearable Posture
  Trainer
☐ White Board

Home Office – Radiation from Wires – Electric Radiation, Magnetic Radiation & Dirty Electricity

☐ Plugged in Bluetooth
  Devices
☐ Plugged in WiFi Devices
☐ Plugged in Wireless
  Devices
☐ Plugged in Smart
  Devices

☐ Air Purifier
☐ Blu-ray DVD Player
☐ Cable Box
☐ Ceiling Fan
☐ Ceiling Lamp with
  Speaker
☐ Ceiling Light Fixture
☐ Ceiling Lights

☐ Charger - Wireless
☐ Chargers
☐ Clock
☐ Cordless Phone
☐ Digital Media Player
☐ Dimmer Switches
☐ DVR
☐ Essential Oil Diffuser
☐ Extension Cords
☐ Fan – Portable
☐ Fax Machine
☐ Fitness Chair -
  Electronic
☐ Fragrance Disseminator
☐ Gaming Systems
☐ HDTV Transmitter

☐ Heater – Portable
☐ Home Air Quality Monitor
☐ Home Audio
☐ Home Devices – Smart
☐ Home Hub for all devices
☐ Home Sensing Carpet
☐ Humidifier – Portable
☐ Internet Streaming Device
☐ Internet TV Device
☐ Internet Video Service
☐ Label Maker
☐ Lamps
☐ Laptop
☐ Light Bulb and Speaker
☐ Light Bulbs – Compact Fluorescent Lights (CFLs)
☐ Light Bulbs – Halogens – Small Base
☐ Light Bulbs – LEDs some
☐ Light Switch
☐ Lighting Systems
☐ Media Streamers
☐ Modem
☐ Motorized Window Blinds
☐ PC Tower

☐ Plug Adaptor/Controller
☐ Power Strips
☐ Printer
☐ Printer – 3D
☐ Projector
☐ Remote Door Bell Chime
☐ Remote Thermostat Sensors
☐ Router
☐ Satellite Receiver
☐ Sauna
☐ Security – Virtual Roommate
☐ Security Camera
☐ Security Lighting
☐ Senior Home Health Monitoring
☐ Signal Booster/Extender
☐ Speakers
☐ Speakers – Smart
☐ Speakers – Wireless
☐ Standalone Streaming Services
☐ Telephone Headset - Wireless
☐ TV
☐ TV Services
☐ Video Game Console
☐ White Board – Electronic

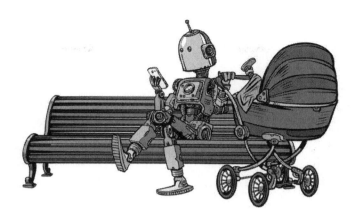

87

Nursery – WiFi/Wireless/Bluetooth/Smart Devices

Some of the below devices can have a WiFi, Wireless, Bluetooth or Smart component in them. Normally there is an interaction with a Smartphone.

☐ Air Filters – Smart
☐ Air Purifier
☐ Alarm Clock sound & vibration
☐ Baby Bottle – Smart
☐ Baby Headset
☐ Baby Heart Rate and Oxygen Monitor
☐ Baby Monitor
☐ Baby Monitor Wrist Band
☐ Baby Projector
☐ Baby Robot
☐ Baby Rocker

☐ Baby Table Lamp – Smart
☐ Baby Temperature and Humidity Device
☐ Baby Vibrating Bed Mat
☐ Baby Wearables
☐ Bassinet or Crib
☐ Bath Water Temperature
☐ Bed
☐ Bed Pad – Smart
☐ Bed Speakers
☐ Bedwetting Alarm

- ☐ Bib – Smart
- ☐ Blanket – Kick-off alert
- ☐ Blu-ray DVD Player
- ☐ Breast Pump
- ☐ Cable Box
- ☐ Ceiling Fan
- ☐ Ceiling Lamp with Speaker
- ☐ Ceiling Light Fixture
- ☐ Cell Phone
- ☐ Charger – Wireless
- ☐ Chargers
- ☐ Child Car Seat
- ☐ Clock
- ☐ Cordless Phone
- ☐ Dancing Robot
- ☐ Diaper – Smart
- ☐ Digital Media Player
- ☐ Dimmer Switches
- ☐ Door Locks
- ☐ DVR
- ☐ eBook Readers
- ☐ EKG Patch
- ☐ Essential Oil Diffuser
- ☐ Fan – Portable
- ☐ Fertility Tracker
- ☐ Fetal Monitor
- ☐ Fetus Camera
- ☐ Fetus Monitoring Band
- ☐ Fragrance Disseminator
- ☐ Glasses – Smart
- ☐ HDTV Transmitter
- ☐ Heater – Portable
- ☐ Home Air Quality Monitor
- ☐ Home Audio
- ☐ Home Automation Item Tracker
- ☐ Home Devices – Smart
- ☐ Home Hub for all devices
- ☐ Home Sensing Carpet
- ☐ Humidifier – Portable
- ☐ Intercom
- ☐ Internet Streaming Device
- ☐ Internet TV Device
- ☐ Internet Video Service
- ☐ iPad/Tablet/Kindle
- ☐ Lamps – Smart
- ☐ Laptop
- ☐ Light Bulb and Speaker
- ☐ Light Bulbs – Smart
- ☐ Light Switch
- ☐ Lighting Systems
- ☐ Mattress Cover – Smart
- ☐ Media Streamers
- ☐ Medical monitoring
- ☐ Motion Detector
- ☐ Motorized Window Blinds
- ☐ MP3 Player
- ☐ Napper & Bouncer – Portable
- ☐ Nursery Environment Monitor

☐ Open or Close Door or Window Sensor
☐ Pacifier – Smart
☐ Plug Adaptor/Controller
☐ Power Strip – Smart
☐ Projector
☐ Remote Door Bell – Chime
☐ Remote Thermostat Sensors
☐ Robot Vacuum
☐ Satellite Receiver
☐ Scale – Baby
☐ Security – Virtual Roommate
☐ Security Camera
☐ Security Lighting
☐ Signal Booster/Extender
☐ Sleep Huggable Pillow
☐ Sleep monitoring System

☐ Sleeping Earphones
☐ Sock – Baby Monitor
☐ Sound Systems
☐ Speakers – Wireless
☐ Speakers – Smart
☐ Spit-up Alert
☐ Standalone Streaming Services
☐ Stroller Speaker
☐ Temperature Monitoring Patch
☐ Thermostat – Smart
☐ TV
☐ TV Services
☐ Video Game Console
☐ Visual Enhancement Glasses
☐ Watch – Smart
☐ Wearable – Baby Monitor

Nursery – Radiation from Wires – Electric Radiation, Magnetic Radiation & Dirty Electricity

☐ Plugged in Bluetooth Devices
☐ Plugged in WiFi Devices
☐ Plugged in Wireless Devices
☐ Plugged in Smart Devices

☐ Air Purifier

☐ Alarm Clock sound & vibration
☐ Baby Monitor
☐ Baby Projector
☐ Baby Robot
☐ Baby Rocker
☐ Baby Table Lamp
☐ Baby Temperature and Humidity Device

☐ Baby Vibrating Bed Mat
☐ Bassinet or Crib
☐ Bed
☐ Bed Pad
☐ Bed Speakers
☐ Bedwetting Alarm
☐ Blu-ray DVD Player
☐ Cable Box
☐ Ceiling Fan
☐ Ceiling Lamp with Speaker
☐ Ceiling Light Fixture
☐ Ceiling Lights
☐ Charger – Wireless
☐ Chargers
☐ Clock
☐ Cordless Phone
☐ Dancing Robot
☐ Digital Media Player
☐ Dimmer Switches
☐ DVR
☐ Electric Bed
☐ Electric Blanket
☐ Essential Oil Diffuser
☐ Extension Cords
☐ Fan – Portable
☐ Fragrance Disseminator
☐ HDTV Transmitter
☐ Heater – Portable
☐ Heating Pad
☐ Home Air Quality Monitor

☐ Home Audio
☐ Home Devices – Smart
☐ Home Hub for all devices
☐ Home Sensing Carpet
☐ Humidifier – Portable
☐ Intercom
☐ Internet Streaming Device
☐ Internet TV Device
☐ Internet Video Service
☐ Lamps
☐ Light Bulb and Speaker
☐ Light Bulbs – Compact Fluorescent Lights (CFLs)
☐ Light Bulbs – Halogens – Small Base
☐ Light Bulbs – LEDs some
☐ Light Switch
☐ Lighting Systems
☐ Mattress Cover
☐ Media Streamers
☐ Medical monitoring
☐ Motion Detector
☐ Motorized Window Blinds
☐ Nursery Environment Monitor
☐ Pacifier – Smart
☐ Plug Adaptor/Controller

- ☐ Power Strips
- ☐ Projector
- ☐ Remote Door Bell Chime
- ☐ Remote Thermostat Sensors
- ☐ Satellite Receiver
- ☐ Scale – Baby
- ☐ Security – Virtual Roommate
- ☐ Security Camera
- ☐ Security Lighting

- ☐ Signal Booster/Extender
- ☐ Smart Home Hub for all devices
- ☐ Sound Systems
- ☐ Speakers
- ☐ Speakers – Smart
- ☐ Standalone Streaming Services
- ☐ TV
- ☐ TV Services
- ☐ Video Game Console

88

Utility Meters – Wireless

- ☐ Utility Meter, Electric
- ☐ Utility Meter, Gas
- ☐ Utility Meter, Water

Utility Meters – Radiation from Wires and Pipes – Electric Radiation, Magnetic Radiation & Dirty Electricity

- ☐ Utility Meter, Electric
- ☐ Utility Meter, Gas
- ☐ Utility Meter, Water

89

Personal/Wearable – WiFi/Wireless/Bluetooth/Smart Devices

Some of the below devices can have a WiFi, Wireless, Bluetooth or Smart component in them. Normally there is an interaction with a Smartphone.

☐ Activity Tracker
☐ Anti-Nausea Band
☐ Back Packs – Smart
☐ Belt – Smart
☐ Brain Activity Tracker
☐ Cell Phone
☐ Child Locator – Wearable
☐ Child's Bone Conduction Headphones
☐ Child's Smartphone Watch
☐ Child's Vital Signs Monitor
☐ Child's Wireless Microphone
☐ Cycling Glasses – Smart
☐ Diabetes Monitor
☐ Earbuds
☐ Ear Piece
☐ Earmuffs
☐ eBook Readers
☐ EEG Monitor
☐ EKG or ECG Monitor
☐ EKG Patch

☐ Fall/Safety Monitoring Lamp
☐ Fertility Monitor
☐ Fetus Camera
☐ Fetus Monitoring Band
☐ Fitness – Wearables
☐ Fitness Coach
☐ Fitness Trackers
☐ Gesture Control Device – Wearable
☐ Glasses – Smart
☐ Glasses – Camera
☐ Gloves for Gaming – Wireless
☐ Head Phones – Wireless
☐ Headband Headset
☐ Health – Wearables
☐ Hearing Aids
☐ Hearing Aid Ear Buds – Bluetooth
☐ Hearing Amplification – Long Range
☐ Hearing Implant inside ear

☐ Heart Rate Sensor
☐ Home Automation Item Tracker
☐ Horseback Rider Fall/Safety Monitor
☐ Intestinal Movement Tracker – Wireless
☐ iPad/Tablet/Kindle
☐ Laptop
☐ Luggage – Smart
☐ Massager – Smart
☐ Media Streamers
☐ Meditation Head Band – Smart
☐ Microphone – Wearable
☐ Migraine – Anti-stimulation
☐ Motion-Ring 3D space Recognition Sensor
☐ MP3 Player
☐ Neckloops
☐ Noise Cancelling Earbuds

☐ Pain Relief – Wearable
☐ Personal Environment Monitor
☐ Respiratory Monitor
☐ Ring – Smart
☐ Senior Home Health Monitoring
☐ Shoe Insole – Smart
☐ Shoes – Smart
☐ Speakers – Baseball Cap
☐ Speakers – Wearable
☐ Stroke Detection Device
☐ Sweat Sensing Monitor
☐ Ultrasound Scanner
☐ Underwear – Smart
☐ Virtual Reality/Augmented Reality Glasses
☐ Visual Enhancement Glasses
☐ Watch – Smart
☐ Wearables – General

Personal/Wearable – Radiation from Wires – Electric Radiation, Magnetic Radiation & Dirty Electricity

☐ Plugged in Bluetooth Devices
☐ Plugged in WiFi Devices

☐ Plugged in Wireless Devices
☐ Plugged in Smart Devices

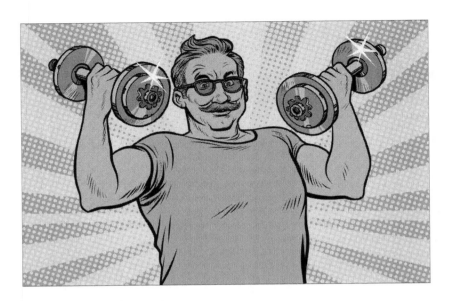

90

Fitness/Exercise/Exercise Room – WiFi/Wireless/ Bluetooth/Smart Devices

Some of the below devices can have a WiFi, Wireless, Bluetooth or Smart component in them. Normally there is an interaction with a Smartphone.

☐ Ab Wheel – Smart
☐ Aerobic Equipment
☐ Air Filters – Smart
☐ Air Purifier
☐ Basketballs – Smart
☐ Belly-Fat Sensor
☐ Bike Airbag Vest
☐ Bike Computer
☐ Bike Helmet – Smart

☐ Bike Stationary – Smart
☐ Bike Tracker
☐ Blu-ray DVD Player
☐ Boxing Punch Tracker
☐ Cable Box
☐ Calorie Intake Monitor
☐ Ceiling Fan
☐ Ceiling Lamp with
   Speaker

☐ Cell Phone
☐ Charger – Wireless
☐ Chargers
☐ Clock
☐ Cordless Phone
☐ Core Equipment – Smart
☐ Cycling Glasses – Smart
☐ Digital Media Player
☐ Dimmer Switches
☐ Door Locks
☐ Drone – Gesture Controlled – Wireless
☐ DVR
☐ Earbuds
☐ eBook Readers
☐ Exercise Equipment
☐ Exercise Hoop – Smart
☐ Fan – Portable
☐ Fitness Coach
☐ Fitness Skin Suit – Smart
☐ Fitness Trackers
☐ Fitness Wearables
☐ Fragrance Disseminator
☐ Gaming Systems
☐ Glasses – Smart
☐ Glove – Smart
☐ Golf Cart Follower – Smart
☐ HDTV Transmitter
☐ Head Phones – Wireless
☐ Headband Headset

☐ Health – Wearables
☐ Heater – Portable
☐ Home Air Quality Monitor
☐ Home Audio
☐ Home Automation Item Tracker
☐ Home Devices – Smart
☐ Home Hub for all devices
☐ Home Sensing Carpet
☐ Humidifier – Portable
☐ Intercom
☐ Internet Streaming Device
☐ Internet TV Device
☐ Internet Video Service
☐ iPad/Tablet/Kindle
☐ Jump Rope – Smart
☐ Laptop
☐ Light Bulb and Speaker
☐ Light Bulbs – Smart
☐ Light Switch
☐ Lighting Systems
☐ Media Streamers
☐ Motion Detector
☐ Motorized Window Blinds
☐ MP3 Player
☐ Neckloops
☐ Open or Closed Door or Window Sensor
☐ Pedometer – Bluetooth

- ☐ Plug Adaptor/Controller
- ☐ Power Strip – Smart
- ☐ Projector
- ☐ Pushup Stands – Smart
- ☐ Remote Thermostat Sensors
- ☐ Resistance Bands – Smart
- ☐ Respiratory Monitor
- ☐ Robot Vacuum
- ☐ Satellite Receiver
- ☐ Sauna
- ☐ Security – Virtual Roommate
- ☐ Security Camera
- ☐ Security Lighting
- ☐ Shoe Insole – Smart
- ☐ Shoes – Smart
- ☐ Signal Booster/Extender
- ☐ Snow Skiing Helmet – Smart
- ☐ Snow Skis – Smart
- ☐ Soccer Ball – Smart
- ☐ Speakers – Wireless

- ☐ Speakers – Smart
- ☐ Standalone Streaming Services
- ☐ Tennis Racket – Smart
- ☐ Thermostat – Smart
- ☐ Thyroid Gland Stimulation – Smart
- ☐ TV
- ☐ TV Services
- ☐ Underwear – Smart
- ☐ Video Game Console
- ☐ Virtual Reality Workout Googles
- ☐ Visual Enhancement Glasses
- ☐ Watch – Smart
- ☐ Water Bottle Speaker – Bluetooth
- ☐ Wearables
- ☐ Weight Lifting Equipment – Smart
- ☐ Yoga Exercise Mat – Smart

Fitness/Exercise Room – Radiation from Wires – Electric Radiation, Magnetic Radiation & Dirty Electricity

☐ Plugged in Bluetooth Devices
☐ Plugged in WiFi Devices
☐ Plugged in Wireless Devices
☐ Plugged in Smart Devices

☐ Air Purifier
☐ Bike Computer
☐ Blu-ray DVD Player
☐ Cable Box
☐ Ceiling Fan
☐ Ceiling Lamp with Speaker
☐ Charger - Wireless
☐ Chargers
☐ Clock
☐ Cordless Phone
☐ Dimmer Switches
☐ DVR
☐ Electric Aerobic Equipment
☐ Electric Core Equipment
☐ Electric Exercise Equipment
☐ Electric Weight Lifting Equipment
☐ Extension Cords

☐ Fan – Portable
☐ Fitness Trackers
☐ Fragrance Disseminator
☐ Gaming Systems
☐ HDTV Transmitter
☐ Heater – Portable
☐ Home Air Quality Monitor
☐ Home Audio
☐ Home Devices – Smart
☐ Home Hub for all devices
☐ Home Sensing Carpet
☐ Humidifier – Portable
☐ Intercom
☐ Internet Streaming Device
☐ Internet TV Device
☐ Internet Video Service
☐ Light Bulb and Speaker
☐ Light Bulbs – Compact Fluorescent Lights (CFLs)
☐ Light Bulbs – Halogens – Small Base
☐ Light Bulbs – LEDs some
☐ Light Switch
☐ Lighting Systems

☐ Media Streamers
☐ Motion Detector
☐ Motorized Window Blinds
☐ Plug Adaptor/Controller
☐ Power Strips
☐ Projector
☐ Remote Thermostat Sensors
☐ Satellite Receiver
☐ Sauna
☐ Security – Virtual Roommate

☐ Security Camera
☐ Security Lighting
☐ Signal Booster/Extender
☐ Smart Home Hub for all devices
☐ Speakers
☐ Speakers – Smart
☐ Standalone Streaming Services
☐ TV
☐ TV Services
☐ Video Game Console
☐ Yoga Exercise Mat

91

Pet – WiFi/Wireless/Bluetooth/Smart Devices

Some of the below devices can have a WiFi, Wireless, Bluetooth or Smart component in them. Normally there is an interaction with a Smartphone.

☐ Cat Exercise Machine Treadmill
☐ Dog Barking Control
☐ Fences
☐ Fish tank – Smart
☐ Pet Activity Monitor
☐ Pet Bed
☐ Pet Camera
☐ Pet Door
☐ Pet Doorbell

☐ Pet Feeder
☐ Pet Food Bowl
☐ Pet Monitoring – Habits and Sleep
☐ Pet Monitoring – Location
☐ Pet Toys
☐ Pet Tracking Camera
☐ Pet Treat Dispenser - WiFi

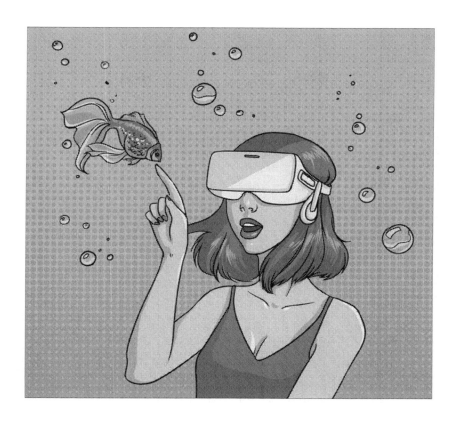

- ☐ Pet Water Bowl
- ☐ Pet Wearable Video Camera
- ☐ Remote Reward Dog Trainer Treats
- ☐ Robot Pet Camera
- ☐ Sliding Glass Pet Door – Smart
- ☐ Smartphone – Dog Trainer

Pet – Radiation from Wires – Electric Radiation, Magnetic Radiation & Dirty Electricity

- ☐ Plugged in Bluetooth Devices
- ☐ Plugged in WiFi Devices
- ☐ Plugged in Wireless Devices
- ☐ Plugged in Smart Devices

92

Kitchen – WiFi/Wireless/Bluetooth/Smart Devices

Some of the below devices can have a WiFi, Wireless, Bluetooth or Smart component in them. Normally there is an interaction with a Smartphone.

☐ Air Filters – Smart
☐ Air Purifier
☐ Baking Scale
☐ Blender
☐ Blu-ray DVD Player
☐ Cable Box
☐ Ceiling Fan
☐ Ceiling Lamp with
   Speaker
☐ Ceiling Light Fixture
☐ Cell Phone
☐ Charger – Wireless
☐ Chargers
☐ Clock
☐ Coffee Maker
☐ Cooking System - Smart
☐ Cordless Phone
☐ Digital Media Player
☐ Dimmer Switches
☐ Dishwasher
☐ Door Locks
☐ DVR
☐ eBook Readers
☐ Essential Oil Diffuser
☐ Fan – Portable

☐ Fragrance Disseminator
☐ Freezer
☐ Frying Pan
☐ Glasses – Smart
☐ HDTV Transmitter
☐ Heater – Portable
☐ Home Air Quality
   Monitor
☐ Home Audio
☐ Home Automation Item
   Tracker
☐ Home Devices – Smart
☐ Home Hub for all
   devices
☐ Hot Water Kettle
☐ Humidifier – Portable
☐ Intercom
☐ Internet Streaming
   Device
☐ Internet TV Device
☐ Internet Video Service
☐ iPad/Tablet/Kindle
☐ Kitchen Scale
☐ Laptop
☐ Light Bulb and Speaker

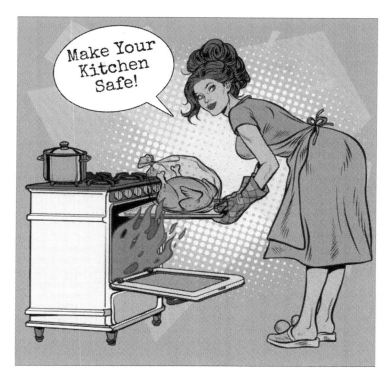

☐ Light Bulbs – Smart
☐ Light Strips – Fluorescent
☐ Light Strips – LEDs
☐ Light Switch
☐ Lighting Systems
☐ Meat Thermometer – Smart
☐ Media Streamers
☐ Microwave Oven
☐ Motion Detector
☐ Motorized Window Blinds
☐ MP3 Player

☐ Open or Close Door or Window Sensor
☐ Plug Adaptor/Controller
☐ Power Strip – Smart
☐ Projector
☐ Refrigerator
☐ Refrigerator Camera
☐ Remote Door Bell Chime
☐ Remote Thermostat Sensors
☐ Robot Vacuum
☐ Satellite Receiver
☐ Security – Virtual Roommate

☐ Security Camera
☐ Security Lighting
☐ Senior Home Health
   Monitoring
☐ Signal Booster/Extender
☐ Slow Cooker
☐ Speakers – Wireless
☐ Speakers – Smart
☐ Standalone Streaming
   Services
☐ Stove
☐ Tea Kettle

☐ Temperature Probe
☐ Thermostat – Smart
☐ TV
☐ TV Services
☐ Video Game Console
☐ Visual Enhancement
   Glasses
☐ Watch – Smart
☐ Water Bottle – Smart
☐ Water Cooking – Smart
☐ Water Filtration System

Kitchen – Radiation from Wires – Electric Radiation, Magnetic Radiation & Dirty Electricity

☐ Plugged in Bluetooth
   Devices
☐ Plugged in WiFi Devices
☐ Plugged in Wireless
   Devices
☐ Plugged in Smart
   Devices
☐ Air Purifier
☐ Baking Scale
☐ Blender
☐ Blu-ray DVD Player
☐ Cable Box
☐ Ceiling Fan
☐ Ceiling Lamp with
   Speaker
☐ Ceiling Light Fixture
☐ Ceiling Lights

☐ Charger - Wireless
☐ Chargers
☐ Clock
☐ Coffee Maker
☐ Cooking System – Smart
☐ Cordless Phone
☐ Digital Media Player
☐ Dimmer Switches
☐ Dishwasher
☐ DVR
☐ Electric Frying Pan
☐ Electric Hot Water
   Kettle
☐ Electric Slow Cooker
☐ Essential Oil Diffuser
☐ Extension Cords
☐ Fan – Portable

☐ Fragrance Disseminator
☐ Freezer
☐ Frying Pan
☐ HDTV Transmitter
☐ Heater – Portable
☐ Home Air Quality Monitor
☐ Home Audio
☐ Home Devices – Smart
☐ Home Hub for all devices
☐ Humidifier
☐ Humidifier – Portable
☐ Intercom
☐ Internet Streaming Device
☐ Internet TV Device
☐ Internet Video Service
☐ Lamps
☐ Light Bulb and Speaker
☐ Light Bulbs – Compact Fluorescent Lights (CFLs)
☐ Light Bulbs – Halogens – Small Base
☐ Light Bulbs – LEDs some
☐ Light Strips – Fluorescent
☐ Light Strips – LEDs
☐ Light Switch
☐ Lighting Systems
☐ Media Streamers
☐ Microwave Oven

☐ Motion Detector
☐ Motorized Window Blinds
☐ Plug Adaptor/Controller
☐ Power Strips
☐ Projector
☐ Refrigerator
☐ Refrigerator Camera
☐ Remote Door Bell Chime
☐ Remote Thermostat Sensors
☐ Satellite Receiver
☐ Security – Virtual Roommate
☐ Security Camera
☐ Security Lighting
☐ Senior Home Health Monitoring
☐ Signal Booster/Extender
☐ Speakers
☐ Speakers – Smart
☐ Standalone Streaming
☐ Stove
☐ Toaster Oven
☐ TV
☐ TV Services
☐ Video Game Console
☐ Visual Enhancement Glasses
☐ Water Cooking – Smart
☐ Water Filtration System, Electric

93

Bathroom – WiFi/Wireless/Bluetooth/Smart Devices

Some of the below devices can have a WiFi, Wireless, Bluetooth or Smart component in them. Normally there is an interaction with a Smartphone.

☐ Air Filters – Smart
☐ Air Purifier
☐ Bathmat – Smart
☐ Bathroom Fan with Speaker
☐ Bathroom Humidity Sensor
☐ Bathroom Speakers
☐ Ceiling Fan
☐ Ceiling Lamp with Speaker
☐ Ceiling Light Fixture
☐ Cell Phone
☐ Charger – Wireless
☐ Chargers
☐ Clock
☐ Dimmer Switches
☐ Door Locks
☐ Earbuds
☐ eBook Readers
☐ Essential Oil Diffuser
☐ Fan – Portable
☐ Fragrance Disseminator
☐ Glasses – Smart
☐ HDTV Transmitter

☐ Head Phones – Wireless
☐ Heater – Portable
☐ Home Air Quality Monitor
☐ Home Audio
☐ Home Automation Item Tracker
☐ Home Devices – Smart
☐ Home Hub for all devices
☐ Humidifier – Portable
☐ Intercom
☐ iPad/Tablet/Kindle
☐ Light Bulb and Speaker
☐ Light Bulbs – Smart
☐ Light Switch
☐ Lighting Systems
☐ Media Streamers
☐ Mirror – Smart
☐ Motion Detector
☐ MP3 Player
☐ Open or Close Door or Window Sensor
☐ Plug Adaptor/Controller
☐ Power Strip – Smart

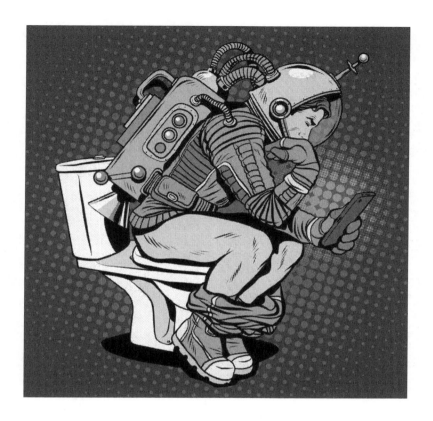

- ☐ Remote Door Bell Chime
- ☐ Remote Thermostat Sensors
- ☐ Robot Vacuum
- ☐ Scale – Adult
- ☐ Scale – Baby
- ☐ Sauna
- ☐ Security Camera
- ☐ Security Lighting
- ☐ Security – Virtual Roommate

- ☐ Senior Home Health Monitoring
- ☐ Signal Booster/Extender
- ☐ Speakers – Wireless
- ☐ Speakers – Smart
- ☐ Thermostat – Smart
- ☐ Toothbrush – Smart
- ☐ Visual Enhancement Glasses

Bathroom — Radiation from Wires — Electric Radiation, Magnetic Radiation & Dirty Electricity

- [ ] Plugged in Bluetooth Devices
- [ ] Plugged in WiFi Devices
- [ ] Plugged in Wireless Devices
- [ ] Plugged in Smart Devices

- [ ] Air Purifier
- [ ] Bathroom Fan with Speaker
- [ ] Bathroom Humidity Sensor
- [ ] Bathroom Speakers
- [ ] Ceiling Fan
- [ ] Ceiling Lamp with Speaker
- [ ] Ceiling Light Fixture
- [ ] Charger — Wireless
- [ ] Chargers
- [ ] Clock
- [ ] Curling Iron
- [ ] Dimmer Switches
- [ ] Electric Shaver
- [ ] Electric Shaver Charger
- [ ] Electric Toothbrush Holder
- [ ] Essential Oil Diffuser
- [ ] Extension Cords
- [ ] Fan — Portable

- [ ] Fragrance Disseminator
- [ ] Hair Dryer
- [ ] HDTV Transmitter
- [ ] Heater — Portable
- [ ] Home Air Quality Monitor
- [ ] Home Audio
- [ ] Home Devices — Smart
- [ ] Home Hub for all devices
- [ ] Humidifier — Portable
- [ ] Intercom
- [ ] Light Bulb and Speaker
- [ ] Light Bulbs — Compact Fluorescent Lights (CFLs)
- [ ] Light Bulbs — Halogens — Small Base
- [ ] Light Bulbs — LEDs some
- [ ] Light Switch
- [ ] Lighted Vanity Mirror
- [ ] Lighting Systems
- [ ] Media Streamers
- [ ] Motion Detector
- [ ] Plug Adaptor/Controller
- [ ] Power Strip
- [ ] Remote Door Bell Chime
- [ ] Remote Thermostat Sensors

☐ Sauna
☐ Security – Virtual
   Roommate
☐ Security Camera
☐ Security Lighting
☐ Senior Home Health
   Monitoring
☐ Signal Booster/Extender

☐ Speakers
☐ Speakers – Smart
   Services
☐ TV
☐ TV Services
☐ Video Game Console
☐ Visual Enhancement
   Glasses

94

Outside/Patio – WiFi/Wireless/Bluetooth/Smart Devices

Some of the below devices can have a WiFi, Wireless, Bluetooth or Smart component in them. Normally there is an interaction with a Smartphone.

☐ Blu-ray DVD Player
☐ Cable Box
☐ Ceiling Fan
☐ Ceiling Lamp with
   Speaker
☐ Ceiling Light Fixture
☐ Cell Phone
☐ Charger – Wireless
☐ Chargers
☐ Clock
☐ Cordless Phone
☐ Delivery Door - Smart
☐ Digital Media Player
☐ Dimmer Switches

☐ Door Bell
☐ Door Locks
☐ DVR
☐ eBook Readers
☐ Essential Oil Diffuser
☐ Fan – Portable
☐ Flower Pot with
   Speakers
☐ Fragrance Disseminator
☐ Gaming Systems
☐ Garden Sensor
☐ Gas Leak Detector
☐ Glasses – Smart
☐ HDTV Transmitter

- ☐ Head Phones – Wireless
- ☐ Heater – Portable
- ☐ Home Audio
- ☐ Home Automation Item Tracker
- ☐ Home Devices – Smart
- ☐ Home Hub for all devices
- ☐ Humidifier – Portable
- ☐ Ice Cooler with Speakers
- ☐ Intelligent Lock Box
- ☐ Intercom
- ☐ Internet Streaming Device
- ☐ Internet TV Device
- ☐ Internet Video Service
- ☐ iPad/Tablet/Kindle
- ☐ Irrigation System
- ☐ Lamps – Smart
- ☐ Laptop
- ☐ Light Bulb and Speaker
- ☐ Light Bulbs – Smart
- ☐ Light Switch
- ☐ Lighting
- ☐ Lighting Systems
- ☐ Meat Thermometer – Smart
- ☐ Media Streamers
- ☐ Medical monitoring
- ☐ Meditation Tracker
- ☐ Microphone
- ☐ Motion Detector
- ☐ MP3 Player
- ☐ Open or Close Door or Window Sensor
- ☐ Outdoor Grill
- ☐ Outdoor Hub
- ☐ Outdoor Lights with Speakers
- ☐ Outdoor Lock
- ☐ Outdoor Motion Detectors
- ☐ Outdoor Smoker
- ☐ Patio Daybed
- ☐ Patio Heater
- ☐ Patio Heater with Speakers
- ☐ Plug Adaptor/Controller
- ☐ Power Strip – Smart
- ☐ Projector
- ☐ Propane Tank Level Monitor
- ☐ Remote Door Bell Chime
- ☐ Remote Thermostat Sensors
- ☐ Satellite Receiver
- ☐ Sauna
- ☐ Security Camera
- ☐ Security Lighting
- ☐ Senior Home Health Monitoring
- ☐ Signal Booster/Extender
- ☐ Speakers – Wireless
- ☐ Speakers – Smart

☐ Speakers in Spa
☐ Standalone Streaming
   Services
☐ Thermostat – Smart
☐ TV
☐ TV Services
☐ Umbrella Speakers
☐ Utility Meter, Electric
☐ Utility Meter, Gas

☐ Utility Meter, Water

☐ Video Game Console
☐ Visual Enhancement
   Glasses
☐ Watch – Smart
☐ Water Bottle – Smart
☐ Water Leak Detector
☐ Weather Station

Outside/Patio – Radiation from Wires – Electric Radiation, Magnetic Radiation & Dirty Electricity

☐ Plugged in Bluetooth
   Devices
☐ Plugged in WiFi Devices
☐ Plugged in Wireless
   Devices
☐ Plugged in Smart
   Devices

☐ Buried Power Lines
☐ Cable TV Line
☐ Overhead Power Lines
☐ Telephone Line
☐ Utility Meter, Electric
☐ Utility Meter, Gas
☐ Utility Meter, Water
☐ Water Line

☐ Blu-ray DVD Player
☐ Cable Box

☐ Cable TV Line
☐ Ceiling Fan
☐ Ceiling Fans
☐ Ceiling Lamp with
   Speaker
☐ Ceiling Light Fixture
☐ Charger – Wireless
☐ Chargers
☐ Clock – Electric
☐ Cordless Phone
☐ Digital Media Player
☐ Dimmer Switches
☐ DVR
☐ Electric Outdoor
   Grill/Smoker
☐ Electric Patio Daybed
☐ Electric Patio Heater
☐ Electric Patio Heater,
   Bluetooth Speakers

☐ Essential Oil Diffuser
☐ Extension Cords
☐ Fan – Portable
☐ Fragrance Disseminator
☐ Gaming Systems
☐ HDTV Transmitter
☐ Heater – Portable
☐ Home Audio
☐ Home Devices – Smart
☐ Home Hub for all devices
☐ Humidifier – Portable
☐ Ice Cooler with Speakers
☐ Intelligent Lock Box
☐ Intercom
☐ Internet Streaming Device
☐ Internet TV Device
☐ Internet Video Service
☐ Irrigation System
☐ Irrigation System Controller
☐ Lamps
☐ Light Bulb and Speaker
☐ Light Bulbs – Compact Fluorescent Lights (CFLs)
☐ Light Bulbs – Halogens – Small Base
☐ Light Bulbs – LEDs some
☐ Light Switch
☐ Lighting

☐ Lighting Systems
☐ Media Streamers
☐ Medical monitoring
☐ Meditation Tracker
☐ Microphone
☐ Motion Detector
☐ Outdoor Grill
☐ Outdoor Hub
☐ Outdoor Lights with Speakers
☐ Outdoor Motion Detectors
☐ Outdoor WiFi Hub
☐ Patio Daybed
☐ Patio Heater
☐ Patio Heater with Speakers
☐ Plug Adaptor/Controller
☐ Power Strip
☐ Projector
☐ Remote Door Bell Chime
☐ Remote Thermostat Sensors
☐ Satellite Receiver
☐ Sauna
☐ Security Camera
☐ Security Lighting
☐ Senior Home Health Monitoring
☐ Signal Booster/Extender
☐ Speakers
☐ Speakers – Smart

☐ Speakers in Spa
☐ Standalone Streaming
  Services
☐ Thermostat

☐ TV
☐ TV Services
☐ Video Game Console
☐ Water Leak Detector

95

Laundry Room – WiFi/Wireless/Bluetooth/Smart Devices

Some of the below devices can have a WiFi, Wireless, Bluetooth or Smart component in them. Normally there is an interaction with a Smartphone.

☐ Air Filters – Smart
☐ Air Purifier
☐ Ceiling Fans
☐ Ceiling Lamp with
  Speaker
☐ Ceiling Light Fixture
☐ Cell Phone
☐ Charger – Wireless
☐ Chargers
☐ Clock
☐ Cordless Phone
☐ Dimmer Switches
☐ Door Locks
☐ Dryer
☐ Fan – Portable
☐ Fragrance Disseminator

☐ HDTV Transmitter
☐ Heater – Portable
☐ Home Air Quality
  Monitor
☐ Home Audio
☐ Home Devices – Smart
☐ Home Hub for all
  devices
☐ Humidifier – Portable
☐ Intercom
☐ Lamps
☐ Light Bulb and Speaker
☐ Light Bulbs – Smart
☐ Light Switch
☐ Lighting
☐ Lighting Systems

☐ Motion Detector
☐ Open or Closed Door or
   Window Sensor
☐ Plug Adaptor/Controller
☐ Remote Door Bell
   Chime
☐ Remote Thermostat
   Sensors
☐ Robot Vacuum
☐ Security Camera

☐ Security Lighting
☐ Security – Virtual
   Roommate
☐ Signal Booster/Extender
☐ Speakers – Wireless
☐ Speakers – Smart
☐ Thermostat – Smart
☐ TV
☐ Washer
☐ Watch – Smart

Laundry Room – Radiation from Wires – Electric Radiation, Magnetic Radiation & Dirty Electricity

☐ Plugged in Bluetooth
   Devices
☐ Plugged in WiFi Devices
☐ Plugged in Wireless
   Devices
☐ Plugged in Smart
   Devices

☐ Air Purifier
☐ Ceiling Fans
☐ Ceiling Lamp with
   Speaker
☐ Ceiling Light Fixture
☐ Charger – Wireless
☐ Chargers
☐ Clock
☐ Cordless Phone
☐ Dimmer Switches
☐ Dryer

☐ Essential Oil Diffuser
☐ Extension Cords
☐ Fan – Portable
☐ Fragrance Disseminator
☐ HDTV Transmitter
☐ Heater – Portable
☐ Home Air Quality
   Monitor
☐ Home Audio
☐ Home Devices – Smart
☐ Home Hub for all
   devices
☐ Humidifier – Portable
☐ Intercom
☐ Lamps
☐ Light Bulb and Speaker
☐ Light Bulbs – Compact
   Fluorescent Lights
   (CFLs)

☐ Light Bulbs – Halogens
   – Small Base
☐ Light Bulbs – LEDs some
☐ Light Switch
☐ Lighting
☐ Lighting Systems
☐ Motion Detector
☐ Plug Adaptor/Controller
☐ Power Strip
☐ Remote Door Bell
   Chime

☐ Remote Thermostat
   Sensors
☐ Security – Virtual
   Roommate
☐ Security Camera
☐ Security Lighting
☐ Signal Booster/Extender
☐ Speakers
☐ Speakers – Smart
☐ TV
☐ Washer

96

Garage/Basement – WiFi/Wireless/Bluetooth/Smart Devices

Some of the below devices can have a WiFi, Wireless, Bluetooth or Smart component in them. Normally there is an interaction with a Smartphone.

☐ Driveway Alert – Smart
☐ Garage Door Opener
☐ Home Audio
☐ Home Devices – Smart
☐ Irrigation Clock
☐ Power Strip – Smart

☐ Sauna
☐ Tools – Smart
☐ Water Filtration System
☐ Water Leak Detector
☐ Water Softener
☐ Weather Station

Garage/Basement – Radiation from Wires – Electric Radiation, Magnetic Radiation & Dirty Electricity

☐ Plugged in Bluetooth Devices
☐ Plugged in WiFi Devices
☐ Plugged in Wireless Devices
☐ Plugged in Smart Devices

☐ Extension Cords
☐ Garage Door Opener
☐ Home Audio
☐ Home Devices – Smart
☐ Irrigation Clock

☐ Light Bulbs – Compact Fluorescent Lights (CFLs)
☐ Light Bulbs – Halogens – Small Base
☐ Light Bulbs – LEDs some
☐ Power Strip
☐ Sauna
☐ Water Filtration System
☐ Water Leak Detector
☐ Water Softener
☐ Weather Station

97

Car – WiFi/Wireless/Bluetooth/Smart Devices

Some of the below devices can have a WiFi, Wireless, Bluetooth or Smart component in them. Normally there is an interaction with a Smartphone.

☐ Advanced Intelligent
    Car Seat Monitoring
☐ Bluetooth Devices
☐ Car License Plate Frame
☐ Car Monitor – Drunk
    and Fatigue Driving
☐ Charger – Wireless

☐ Glasses – Smart
☐ MP3 Player
☐ Smart Devices
☐ Visor Speaker
☐ Watch – Smart
☐ WiFi Devices
☐ Wireless Devices

Car – Radiation from Wires – Electric Radiation, Magnetic Radiation & Dirty Electricity

☐ Anything you plug into a 2-prong or 3-prong adaptor in a car – 120 Volt Devices

98

Equine Devices

Some of the below devices can have a WiFi, Wireless, Bluetooth or Smart component in them. Normally there is an interaction with a Smartphone.

☐ Horse Saddle Movement Monitor
☐ Horseback Rider Fall/Safety Monitor
☐ Wireless Fences

99

Free EMF Consultation

Request a Free 15-minute EMF Consultation.
Contact: www.StopDirtyElectricity.com

Websites & Resources

There are hundreds of fabulous EMF websites. Here are a few of my favorites to get you started.

StopDirtyElectricity.com: Bill Cadwallader, Certified Electromagnetic Radiation Specialist, detects and reduces the electromagnetic radiation threats to your workplace, school, and home. Bill is recognized as an international EMF and 5G expert. https://stopdirtyelectricity.com

Antenna Search: Type your address in the search box and see how many cell towers are in your neighborhood within a two-mile radius. http://www.antennasearch.com

BioInitiative Report (updated 2020) has gathered thousands of peer-reviewed published literature documenting the biological effects of EMFs on human health and the environment. https://bioinitiative.org

Building Biology Institute offers educational courses (and certification) in technical knowledge and practical remediation of electromagnetic radiation. https://buildingbiologyinstitute.org/ To find a Certified Electromagnetic Radiation Specialist in your area go to: https://buildingbiologyinstitute.org/find-an-expert/

Canadians for Safe Technology (C4ST) seeks to educate and inform Canadians and their policy makers about the dangers of the exposures to unsafe levels of radiation from technology, and to work with all levels of government to create healthier communities for children and families across Canada. http://c4st.org

Cell Phone Task Force provides a global clearinghouse for information about wireless technology's injurious effects, and a national support network for people injured or disabled by electromagnetic fields. https://www.cellphonetaskforce.org

CEP (Center for Electro-smog Prevention) is a group dedicated to the purpose of preventing and reducing environmental electromagnetic pollution in California. http://www.electrosmogprevention.org/stop-5g-action-plan/10-actions-to-help-stop-5g/

Create Healthy Homes: Oram Miller is one of the world's leading experts on electromagnetic radiation and 5G. This website provides some of the technical details behind the technology. Createhealthyhomes.com

Electric Sense: This website offers help for those who have EHS (Electromagnetic Hypersensitivity). Lloyd Burrell has interviewed hundreds of scientists, researchers, and health professionals and makes these available via podcasts and videos. This website also includes controversial topics related to 5G, collusion and cover-up, surveillance, etc. https://www.electricsense.com

Environmental Health Trust: Its mission is to safeguard human health and the environment by empowering people with state-of-the-art information. This site keeps up with the latest scientific research and provides a lot of useful tools to use at the grassroots level. https://ehtrust.org

Generation Zapped: This documentary film investigates the potential dangers of prolonged exposure to Radio Frequencies (RF) from wireless technology and its effects on our health and well-being, as well as the health and development of our children. https://generationzapped.com

GUARDS (Global Union Against Radiation Deployment from Space) is an international coalition of scientists speaking out about the environmental hazards of the proliferation of wireless technology and the deployment of 5G satellites. http://www.stopglobalwifi.org

International Appeal to Stop 5G on Earth and in Space. This site deals with environmental issues of technology. https://www.5gspaceappeal.org/the-appeal

International EMF Scientist Appeal: It serves as a credible and influential voice from EMF scientists who are urgently calling upon the United Nations and its sub-organizations, the WHO and UNEP, and all U.N. Member States, for greater health protection on EMF exposure. https://emfscientist.org

Manhattan Neighbors for Safer Telecommunications: Its mission is to bring awareness to the harmful physical and mental health effects of cell phones, Wi-Fi, wireless computer equipment, portable phones, excessive screen time, too-early technology use, wireless utility equipment, and neighborhood cell towers and antennas. https://manhattanneighbors.org

Stop the Assault on Hawaii: A coalition of educated, concerned residents of the Hawaiian islands who have joined in the global effort to limit and/or stop harmful wireless technologies (including 5G and smart meters) from being deployed in our precious islands. http://keepyourpower.org

Take Back Your Power: This group examines the dangers of "smart meters" to your privacy, your health, and your freedom. You can stream the documentary film "Take Back Your Power" for free. https://www.takebackyourpower.net

WATE (We Are The Evidence) intends to expose the suppressed epidemic of sickness, suffering and human rights crisis created by wireless technology radiation; elevate the voice of those injured; defend and secure their rights and compel society and governments to take corrective actions and inform the public of the harm. We work through education, lobbying and legal action. https://wearetheevidence.org

Want more?

EXPOSED: The Electronic Sickening of America and How to Protect Yourself — Includes dangers of 5G & Smart Devices. This book includes references to more than 300 books, articles, and websites related to electromagnetic radiation as well as expanded solutions. www.StopDirtyElectricity.com

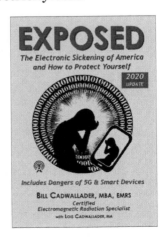

About the Authors

Lois Cadwallader, MA, has been a professional educator all of her adult life.

She is the co-author of the book, *Exposed: The Electronic Sickening of America and How to Protect Yourself – Includes Dangers of 5G & Smart Devices*.

She is a featured writer for Lloyd Burrell's EMF website, www.electricsense.com.

She enjoys hiking, cycling, and volunteering in after-school Good News Clubs®.

Her husband, Bill Cadwallader, MBA, EMRS, is a Certified Electromagnetic Radiation Specialist and served as the technical consultant for this book.

He is the author of *Exposed*, and offers EMF home inspections and remediation in Nevada, Southern California, Southern Utah, and Arizona. He is also available for speaking engagements and phone consultation.

They live in Las Vegas, Nevada, with a 20-year-old cat, "Pushy."

Special acknowledgement to Erin Calkins, Graphic Image and Social Media Consultant, who keeps things youthful and a little edgy. https://www.dramaticrabbit.com

Made in the USA
San Bernardino, CA
31 May 2020

LIVING
BACKWARD

THE *Gift* OF HINDSIGHT IN BUILDING
A TRULY SIGNIFICANT LIFE

ANGELIQUE COOPER MCGLOTTEN

Living Backward
Published by Almond Blossom Media
Copyright © 2015 by Angelique Cooper McGlotten

This title is also available as an Almond Blossom Media e-book.
Visit the author's website: www.livingbackward.com.

Requests for information should be addressed to:
Almond Blossom Media, LLC, 7286 Earlys Road, Warrenton, VA 20187

Developmental Editor: Melissa Wuske
Copyedited, Proofread, and Designed by Girl Friday Productions
Cover Design: Paul Barrett
www.girlfridayproductions.com

ISBN-13: 9780996454919
ISBN-10: 0996454918
e-ISBN: 9780996454902
Library of Congress Control Number: 2015910374

First Edition

Printed in the United States of America

To the gems God has graciously given me the sacred trust and privilege to raise and nurture:

Jared Pierce
Jordan Cayce
Chayil Joie

My heart overflows with joy because of the indescribable ways that you've blessed and continue to bless me! For many years, I've deeply desired to pass on to you a written account of what God has taught me and what His gracious hand upon my life has wrought. This book—part and parcel of my legacy—has allowed me to do just that. It is your momma's gift to you. I pray each of you will resolve to live backward, boldly and unreservedly honoring the Lord with your lives. As you do, may God Almighty continually weave the threads of His unending love, mercy, and grace into the fabric of your consecrated lives. Beautiful, for sure, will the resulting tapestry be— ever and forever magnifying His great and glorious name.

CONTENTS

....

One thing have I asked of the LORD,
that will I seek after:
that I may dwell in the house of the LORD
all the days of my life,
to gaze upon the beauty of the LORD
and to inquire in his temple.
Psalm 27:4

Be exalted, O God, above the heavens!
Let your glory be all over the earth!
Psalm 57:5

Then Jesus told his disciples, "If anyone would come after me, let him deny himself and take up his cross and follow me. For whoever would save his life will lose it, but whoever loses his life for my sake will find it. For what will it profit a man if he gains the whole world and forfeits his soul? Or what shall a man give in return for his soul? For the Son of Man is going to come with his angels in the glory of his Father, and then he will repay each person according to what he has done."
Matthew 16:24–27

INTRODUCTION

··

This past summer, my husband (who is fond of surprises) planned a spontaneous family trip to Canada. We had to spill the beans to our eldest, as he needed to arrange time off work. But our younger son and daughter had no clue until they got into the car and discovered their packed bags in the trunk. We took off from our abode in Virginia, excited about this special time together as a family. In the span of less than five days, we drove well over two thousand miles. After visiting Niagara Falls, we headed over the US border into Ontario. From there we headed to Montreal and then Quebec City. For the second-to-last leg of our trip, my husband planned to take us as far north as New Brunswick. Because it was much farther away, we started the drive late at night.

Three hours into the trip, we stopped for a restroom break at McDonald's. As I settled back into the car, my husband was intently studying the map. He looked over at me and sighed as he started the car. "Honey, I misread the map." Since we were in a foreign country and without an active GPS, we had driven more than 180 miles on the *wrong side of the river.*

From where we were, there was absolutely no way of reaching New Brunswick without crossing the river. Making matters worse, there was no way to cut over to the other side. So we had to drive three hours in the opposite direction back to Quebec City, then travel another four hours up the correct side of the river. Instead of arriving at our hotel at two in the morning as planned, we got there just after nine, exhausted from the long trip.

Later, as I reflected on this incident, it reminded me of my life. When I was thirty-five, my life was great. Blessed with a wonderful husband, two adorable little boys, as well as a nice home, I felt I had gotten my life into place. Naturally, I felt very satisfied. During this period, my husband and I believed that the path we were on and the choices we were making would get us to where we wanted to be. Things seemed to be going quite well until I found myself in the McFrustrated parking lot of life—while everything in my life seemed and looked right, everything wasn't. Although I desired to please God, I lacked a full biblical understanding of His purpose for my life. As a result, I had been going through life conveniently blending what *seemed right for me*—my own ambitions and self-centered desires—with my limited knowledge of what *God desired of me*. I eventually ended up feeling stagnant in my spiritual growth and unfulfilled. Never quite able to connect the dots in my faith walk, I, nonetheless, realized that something was definitely missing. I remember repeatedly saying to myself, *There's got to be more to life than this.* Deep down I knew that Christ died for me to have a life far better than what I was actually experiencing.

Similar to our misadventure in Canada, my husband and I for a long time had thought we were following God's path for our lives. But in reality, we were not fully seeking God's directions. Just like my husband's wrong turn could never have gotten us to where we wanted to go, it finally dawned on me that I could never achieve God's eternal plan for my life if I continued on the path that I was pursuing. In the same way that we made the choice to change direction and get on the right Canadian highway, I needed to change the direction I was headed if I wanted God's best for my life. I'm thankful beyond words that I did.

Each of us is on a path that is taking us *somewhere*. What path are you walking? Where are you today as you come to this book? Maybe you're searching for the right path. Or maybe you realize that the path you're on isn't getting you nearer to where you want to be. Maybe you haven't given much thought to where you're headed. Or maybe you do recognize that you are not on God's path for your life. Regardless of which camp you find yourself in, take heart. It's never too late to discover God's path. No matter where you begin, you can grow in your relationship with God and start seeking His direction. You have not come across this book by accident or chance; you are reading it by God's sovereign design. I've prayed that God's gift of encouragement to me and the things He has taught me would bless you.

God extends to each of us the same gracious invitation that He offered the Israelites long ago: "This is what the LORD says: 'Stop at the crossroads and look around. Ask for the old, godly way, and walk in it. Travel its path, and you will find rest for your souls'" (Jeremiah 6:16, New Living Translation). This good way (as another translation refers to it) is in contrast to the path of our self-empowered choosing. Therefore, we can heed this verse only after we've acknowledged that the road of life traveled without God's guidance leads to a dead end. It results in a fruitless, empty, and ultimately bankrupt life. Indeed, this is the opposite of the purposeful and fulfilling lives that we desperately yearn for and that God zealously desires us to have.

C. S. Lewis wisely said, "We all want progress. But progress is getting nearer to where you want to be. And if you've taken a wrong [turn], then to go forward doesn't get you any nearer."[1] So I pray you will choose to say, *Lord, I desire to walk in the good way! I desire the path that is pleasing to You and that leads to my greatest good.* But I've discovered that many sincere followers of Christ have the same struggle I once had. Namely, how do I practically walk out God's plan for my life? What does a Christ-exalting life look like? How do I grow from who I am into the person God created me to be? And how do I go about building a life that really matters? My purpose in writing this book is to address these very important questions.

---

1. C. S. Lewis, *Mere Christianity* (New York: HarperCollins, 2003), 28.

I remember what it was like to read book after book—some biblically sound and some not so much—in my earnest attempt to live a life pleasing to God. I could never seem to figure out how all the advice and directives in the books fit together. After reading hundreds of books on all aspects of the Christian life, I was finally able to gain a solid biblical understanding of God's eternal purpose for me and how to live what I learned. Little did I realize that during this reading marathon, God had planted a seed of compassion in me that had begun to germinate. Three years ago, the seed began to grow. I became burdened for those whose lives are in disarray because they don't fully understand the true purpose for why they exist. It saddens me that so many of God's sons and daughters are scrounging up the crumbs off the floor when He has invited us to feast at His lavish banquet and to drink deeply from His fountain of love. If we can scarcely imagine the children of an earthly king eating scraps from the floor, then we can't possibly fathom how much this reality must break our Father's heart. Even more, my heart aches that so many of God's people don't really know Him, nor have they truly tasted and seen that He is good (see Psalm 34:8) and infinitely worthy of our lives bringing Him honor and glory.

Out of this heartache, God birthed the desire to write this book: a discipleship tool that condenses into *one* volume those major topics and key principles a person needs to know and understand in order to fulfill God's purpose for creating us. Drawing on God's Word, my spiritual journey and experience, as well as the wisdom and knowledge gleaned from my extensive reading, I wanted to help others connect the dots in their own lives without having to pore through so many books. I want *you* to be able to read one book—*this book*—and come away with a solid understanding of how to live an authentic and purposeful Christ-honoring life. If you're not a follower of Christ and are reading this book out of sheer curiosity, perhaps hoping you can be good enough on your own to get by, I pray that this book will illumine this truth: a life lived apart from God is utterly meaningless. Jesus emphatically declared, "I am the way, and the truth, and the life. No one comes to the Father except through me" (John 14:6). In other words, once we've by faith accepted Jesus's sacrifice on our behalf to erase the debt that God justly demands for our sins, we can be reconciled to God. If you've never before accepted this incredible invitation, God invites you to come just as you are to place your trust in Jesus as your Savior and Redeemer; contrary to common thinking, you don't have to get yourself right first because, in fact, you can't. No matter where you are, at this very moment God desires a personal relationship with you. If you fall into this category, my goal is that, by the time you're done reading this book, you've also gained a coherent biblical worldview. One that perhaps will not only sweetly compel you to follow Jesus Christ but also undergird you as you navigate the myriad complexities of life.

Here's the crux of the matter: although we greatly matter *to* God, God desires us to greatly matter *for* Him. We matter for God when we seek to glorify Him by following the example of Christ. In other words, what ultimately matters in this life—our overarching purpose— is becoming more like Christ in each and every area of our lives, be it as a wife, son, mother, daughter, father, nurse, teacher, athlete, businessman, etc. We have one temporal life to live. When we choose to live it for God's glory and pleasure, the character we forge and what we make of our lives can take on the enduring quality of gold and have value and significance beyond our earthly years. Why chase after mere earthly importance or settle for the allurements of this world—that are both fleeting and short-lived—when what we pursue in this life can count for all eternity? The profound reality that we each can live in such a way that magnifies God's glory *and* simultaneously enriches our own eternal futures is the consuming passion of my life.

Have you ever encountered a massive traffic jam and then turned around to go back in the opposite direction in order to take a different route? Whenever I've done that, something in me wishes I could alert the people in oncoming cars—who haven't yet hit the traffic—about what's up ahead. In regards to life, I hope that this book does something similar.

Wherever you are in your spiritual journey, young or not so young, this book was written with you in mind. It's written plainly enough for the newest follower of Christ to understand yet contains spiritual "meat and potatoes" that will inspire and challenge even a seasoned disciple. Get excited. I believe you've come to this book yearning for more, and here you'll find a road map to help you pursue and reclaim what matters most.

This is not another informational book. Rather, I've used word pictures, analogies, and personal anecdotes to illustrate or highlight important biblical truths. I hope these insights will facilitate what I call head-to-heart understanding: we must first internalize key biblical concepts and principles before we can derive the benefit of their life-changing power.

As we begin this journey, I want you to know that my acceptance of God's invitation to pursue the good way has filled my life with joy, peace, victory, contentment, and meaning—those very things that point to true spiritual progress yet had eluded me for so long. Pursuing this God-centered path has also ignited a passion in me to *live backward* in order to truly *move forward* into building a life of true significance. I pray the same for you.

We commonly use GPS to help us get to where we want to go. It works based on a reverse principle—starting at the intended destination, it works backward to one's current location, factoring in such variables as traffic and construction to provide the best possible route. However, there are times when it accidentally causes us to go in the wrong direction, get turned around, or completely lose our way.

There's another GPS, an infinitely more superior one—God's Positioning System. We don't ever have to plug in our current location, as it knows exactly where each of us is at any given moment. Always perfectly accurate, it will never lead us in the wrong direction or to the wrong destination; with it we ultimately can never lose our way. That's because the omniscient God of the universe has already mapped out the best possible route for each of our lives. He knows the end from the beginning and everything in between concerning each of us; He also knows every possible detour and wrong turn we could ever take. Even when we've gone off course thinking we're in His will, God can—and will—mercifully get us back on track. Just how an active GPS persistently reroutes us after each wrong turn we make, God will continually redirect us to where He wants us to be, provided our heart's desire is to truly follow Him. God is unchanging and His Word is enduring. Therefore, we can have the utmost confidence in His unfailing love and His unwavering promise to lead us and guide us. Starting now we can leave our past—failures, painful memories, shattered dreams, accidents, wrong turns, and detours—in His kind hands, which are absolutely capable of redeeming them all.

If we want to make genuine spiritual progress—avoiding wrong turns and walking in all that God desires for us—we must daily plug into the divine GPS and look to it for direction. Informed and guided by it, our lives will truly matter for God.

Stick with me to the end. I assure you that, besides laying a solid foundation, cultivating the five principles in this book will provide the brick and mortar for you to build and uphold the edifice of a truly significant life—one that ultimately counts in God's estimation.

Deep down, you desire nothing less.

Soli Deo gloria! Glory to God alone!

Blessings,

May 2015
Warrenton, VA

PRINCIPLE 1

·····································

UNDERSTAND TRUE SIGNIFICANCE

CHAPTER 1

······················

IN PURSUIT OF WHAT MATTERS MOST

He is no fool who gives what he cannot keep
to gain that which he cannot lose.
—Jim Elliot (emphasis mine)

You're about to embark on a life-transforming journey. However, I want to emphasize that contrary to popular self-help books, humanistic teachings, New Age ideas, and the like, God, not ourselves, must be the reference point if we desire to live meaningful and significant lives. (If you've skipped over the introduction to jump into the meat of the book, I strongly encourage you to go back and read it.) God has given us the Bible, His Word, so that we may know Him, understand why He created us, and then align our lives accordingly. Yet it's so easy to fall into a flowery version of Christianity where we view God as a cosmic genie who exists to give us what we think will make us happy: a stress-free life, a great career, a picture-perfect home, all the money we could ever need, abs of steel, and so on. However, God does not exist for us; we exist for God.

So as we consider the sweeping idea of living a life of true significance, we must first recognize that the eternal God who created us—along with the sun, moon, billions of stars, galaxies, and everything in the entire universe—is incomprehensibly great and beyond description (see Psalms 71:19, 90:2, 139:6, 145:3, 147:5; Isaiah 55:8–9; Romans 11:33). He is so awesome and infinite that we will never fully understand Him, though, for all eternity, we will continue to increase our knowledge of who He is. Thankfully, God has not created us and then left us to ourselves. Rather, He has chosen to be intimately involved in our lives: He is our Sustainer, Provider, Counselor, and the Lover of our souls, to name a few of His redemptive attributes. God calls us to live for His good pleasure and proclaim the excellence of His great name (see Revelations 4:11; 1 Peter 2:9). Therefore, we magnify God's greatness when we lead lives that reflect His image or point to Him. In fact, though it's an uncommon teaching, God's passion for His own glory is the fundamental reason that He desires us to lead fulfilling lives, lives that honor Him.

Of course, this is not to say that God doesn't want us to lead significant lives for our own benefit. Indeed, He does (see John 10:10). We experience this fulfillment daily as we embrace those things that God has ordained to give our lives meaning. This fulfillment, however, should not be confused with the biblical teaching that, as disciples, our fundamental identity is found in our relationship with Christ; ultimately, our sense of significance is rooted in the fact that we belong to God—we are treasured because He calls us His own. So when I speak of significance or fulfillment in this book, I'm not referring to our positional standing with Christ, for this has already been accomplished through His sacrifice on the cross and nothing more can be added (see Ephesians 2:6). Rather, I'm referring to the outworking of God's eternal purpose for our redeemed yet imperfect lives.

Contrary to our cultural definitions of greatness and success, you don't have to be an incredibly savvy businesswoman, a charismatic leader, a gifted athlete or actress, an innovative philanthropist, or anything of the sort to be great. *Anyone* can be great in God's estimation! As a matter of fact, the desire deeply embedded within each of us to matter and feel significant is not wrong or even unbiblical. The truth is that we should earnestly desire for our lives to be great in God's eyes as we love and serve Him and love and serve others (see Matthew 20:26, 23:11, 37–40, Luke 22:26). However, we must never lose sight that, ultimately, God wants our lives to display His own glory.

GOD'S RENOWN

You may now be wondering: Why does God care so much about His own glory? Isn't it arrogant of God to desire praise for Himself? These are good questions, and we must go to Scripture for the answers. God is impassioned for His glory or honor because having created all things, He and He alone is worthy to receive glory (see Revelations 4:11). This truth is plainly taught in Isaiah 42:8, where God declares, "I am the Lord; that is my name; my glory I give to no other, nor my praise to carved idols." God echoes the same thought in Isaiah 48:11: "how should my name be profaned? My glory I will not give to another." Moving beyond God's own words, Psalm 29:1–2 reveals God's desire for His people to magnify Him: "ascribe to the Lord glory and strength. Ascribe to the Lord the glory due His name." These are but three of many biblical passages where we see God's zeal for His glory.

Moreover, God's renown is integral to His character. His greatness is as much a part of Him as His love or faithfulness, and like His love or faithfulness, He can't help but express it—it can't be suppressed. Therefore, God desires His glory to be displayed just as passionately as He does all His other attributes such as His mercy, justice, compassion, holiness, and omniscience. Indeed, all of God's creation is intended for the grand display of His infinite power, wisdom, and majesty so that "the earth will be filled with knowledge of the glory of the Lord as the waters cover the sea" (Habakkuk 2:14; see also 1 Chronicles 16:9–10, 29; Psalm 108:5, 115:1; Romans 11:36).

The Bible reveals that nothing transcends God's desire for the display of His own glory. This is true for the simple reason that there is nothing or no one higher than God. Because His honor is of supreme importance to Him, God acts for His name's sake no matter the circumstance (see Isaiah 48:9; Ezekiel 20:9, 14, 22, 44). From the Old Testament to the New, all of Scripture confirms that everything the sovereign God of the universe does or allows is to exalt His glory, that the infinite worth of His name may be praised, revered, and adored. In fact, even our salvation was ultimately effected to magnify God's glory (see Isaiah 43:2, 5).

Despite these teachings, we still find it hard to grasp God's passion for His own glory. We have a difficult time reconciling a God who is supposed to be holy—and therefore, not arrogant—with a God who desires His own praise, as this flies in the face of how we view humility. Hence, we are all too easily taken aback or offended by this dichotomous aspect of God's nature. I've discovered that understanding why God wants what He wants is at the heart of change: God desires us to live for His glory because He not only wants the best for us, He also knows what is best for us, as He is all-wise and all-knowing (see Job 12:13; Psalm 147:5; Isaiah 40:28; and Romans 11:33). The great news is that by His sovereign design, anything that glorifies God ultimately serves our greatest interest as well. That's because God Himself is the eternal, unending overflow of all that is pure, holy, virtuous, and beautiful. He is the gracious Giver of everything good and the perfection of all that we long for or desire. He is truly more than all that we could ever need. Therefore, when we purpose to live for His honor and fame, we're simultaneously pursuing our greatest joy and satisfaction. John Piper says it well: "God is most glorified in me when I am most satisfied in Him."[2] As we live our lives to bring joy to our heavenly Father, we discover not only our greatest fulfillment, but we also appropriate more and more of all that He desires for us in Jesus. This is a truth to rejoice in.

---

2.   John Piper, *Desiring God* (Multnomah Books, 2003), 10.

This foundational understanding of God's unbridled passion for His glory means that, although it may otherwise have caught us by surprise, it is God Himself who most desires significance. The following Scriptures underscore this fact: "Let the one who boasts, boast in the Lord" (2 Corinthians 10:17); "The Lord is great and greatly to be praised" (Psalm 96:4); "Let not the wise man boast of his wisdom or the strong man boast of His strength or the rich man boasts of his riches, but let him who boasts, boast in this: that He knows Me" (Jeremiah 9:23–24); "May [we] never boast except in the cross of our Lord Jesus Christ, through which the world has been crucified to [us], and [us] to the world" (Galatians 6:14). These verses inherently teach that because God is good, holy, and righteous, only He can rightly or flawlessly desire His own self-importance, which is not to be confused with human vanity. Each also asserts God's zeal to seek from His people the superlative honor He is rightly due—the essence of true worship.

Nevertheless, we make much more ado about ourselves than we do about God because our default is to act counter to His will. It's critical we understand that though we are made in God's image (see Genesis 1:26–27), we are, in a sense, but specks compared to Him. Therefore, our deep yearning to matter and make a name for ourselves is like a drop in the bucket—no, more like a drop in a lake—compared to the endless ocean of God's rightful desire to be made much of. This picture has deepened my appreciation of God's passion for His glory.

How humbling, then, that a primary way God desires to display His glory is through His people. That God has given us such an incredible privilege is an unfathomable wonder. We are truly the bearers of His image, created to reflect the light of His glory in this dark and fallen world filled with broken and hopeless people who desperately need to know Him. Practically speaking, God desires us to continually seek Him and invite Him into each and every thing that we do. In essence, He requests that our desire to matter be wrapped or hidden in His zeal to bring glory to Himself.

THE TIME FACTOR

You've likely heard the inspiring poem called "The Dash" by Linda Ellis—you're born, you die, and the dash is what happens in between. You've also probably heard the maxim: "Time marches on." While we know deep down that time waits for no one, we, nevertheless, tend to go through life as though time is on our side. We also tend to forget that the dash is our one and only opportunity to make our mark on eternity. Doubtless, Satan—our archenemy, who seduced our first parents, Adam and Eve, to disobey God (see Genesis 3)—also deceives us into thinking that we have plenty of time. But life is fragile and uncertain. James 4:14 clearly teaches, "Yet you do not know what your life will be like tomorrow. You are *just* a vapor that appears for a little while and then vanishes away" (New American Standard Bible). Like a flower that is here today and gone tomorrow, so is the brevity of our lives (see 1 Peter 1:24). Therefore, a forward perspective of time marching on leads to a subtle but grave pitfall: it predisposes us to put off leading purposeful lives *precisely because we assume we have time on our side.* This is to our peril, and it's bolstered by the fact that there's something primal in us that seeks to avoid pondering our own mortality.

The issue is not that we don't ever consider our death, but rather that we don't value enough the preciousness of time. In fact, numerous findings suggest that neither mortality nor imminent death is the primary reason that some people experience a midlife crisis.[3] Rather, people experience a midlife crisis because it's as if they are suddenly confronted by the reality that time has somehow passed them by, and they aren't where they thought they'd be. Thankfully, however, with God's Word we each can renew our minds and be fruitful, no matter our age (see Romans 12:2; Psalm 92:14). The title of this book hints at

---

3. Susan S. Lang, "Crisis or just stress?" *Cornell Chronicle* (March 19, 2001): http://news.cornell.edu/stories/2001/03/midlife-crisis-less-common-many-believe (accessed June 14, 2014).

this truth. Since the idea of living backward is counterintuitive, let's delve into what it means.

TICKING DOWN . . .

The concept of living backward is meant to counter this grave mind-set that we have time on our hands. Time is truly priceless—once it's gone, you can never get it back. Because time is an invaluable commodity, I want to challenge you to reorient your thinking. I hope you'll embrace a paradigm shift and begin to view your time on earth not as simply marching forward but as elapsing. Yes, do enjoy and celebrate each and every year with which God blesses you. But I want you to truly grasp that with each passing year you haven't just *gained* another birthday or more time to live—you've also *lost* more of the precious, irretrievable time that you have been allotted to create significance in your life. To varying degrees, each of us has already lost or squandered countless opportunities to endow our lives with true significance, because contrary to the world's system, not everything "great" that we do in this life will leave a mark on eternity. Indeed, many of these things absolutely won't.

As much as we may want to minimize this fact, each of our lives is much like a fully wound clock that is steadily ticking down. Ticking down to that eventful and inescapable moment in the future—God's final assessment of our lives. Since Scripture teaches that this evaluation will have sweeping ramifications for all eternity, it's of the utmost importance to heed this counsel and engage life with an eternal mind-set. Yet we generally don't stop to consider our lives—much less how fleeting they are—within the context of our earthly time clock winding down, only to be recalibrated for time without end.

LIVING BACKWARD

But how exactly do we live backward? First, we must keenly recognize that when we stand before God (even free of condemnation as His redeemed), our vain, self-centered accomplishments will never meet His criteria for true greatness and enduring significance. Second, we must grasp that the ramifications of God's assessment of our lives are profound: not only is the quality of our eternal existence—rewards, losses, treasures, forfeitures, commendations, and degree of responsibilities—at stake, but more importantly, so is the display of God's glory in our lives (see Jeremiah 17:10; 2 Corinthians 5:10). Therefore, we must start to weigh everything against the sobering reality that (aside from salvation which cannot be earned) the quality of our future eternal existence is predicated upon the everyday choices that we make in the here and now.

To live backward, then, is to intentionally live as though every tick—or choice—you make *now* matters *forever*. Like the saying, "Begin with the end in mind," living backward is to chart the course of our lives using the reverse orientation employed by GPS. Our destination is that decisive moment in the future when God evaluates what we each have made of our lives. Using this as our reference point we then work backward, engaging life through the lens of time elapsing, not accruing, in order to wisely redeem the limited time God has designated to each of us before we reach our "final destination"—for then it will be too late to weave significance into our lives. Many of us have not apprehended the all-encompassing need to prepare ourselves for this momentous day. Embracing the gift of hindsight changes that.

I've heard eternity described as a line extending forever with no end; relative to eternity our lives are but a teeny, tiny dot on that line. Yet we focus on and live for the dot, forgetting that it's the endless line that really matters. Consequently, many of us give little or no thought to either our forever existence or Jesus's command to store up treasures above and not on the earth. By default, then, many of us are absorbed in the things of this world. Yet we can't idly live for ourselves and please God. These desires simply cannot coexist. My hope is that embracing a reverse perspective of time will enable us to more deeply appreciate that this temporal life is but a vanishing mist relative to eternity. And that, in turn, we'll begin to make steady progress toward living purposefully, both to showcase God's glory and for our greatest eternal good.

THE FS FACTOR VS. THE EV FACTOR

Now that we know what it means to live backward, how do we start? By taking honest inventory of our lives and asking some hard questions: What am I really building with my life? Does God care about the things in which I'm investing time, energy, and money? Am I seeking to bear fruit such as love, patience, self-control (see Galatians 5:22), and reflect the light of Christ in this dark world? Are my goals and activities advancing God's kingdom, or am I preoccupied building my own? How much of what I'm busy doing and pursuing will endure after I've exited this earthly life? In essence, am I living for what ultimately matters? The truth is there's a world of difference between a successful life and a significant life. We must acknowledge that it is not large bank accounts or stock holdings, nor status symbols—fashion accessories, luxury vehicles, boats, time-share destinations, luxurious homes, prized paintings, prestigious schools attended by the children God has entrusted to us—nor great occupations, nor titles, nor socioeconomic standing, nor popularity, nor opinions and the like, that give our lives true meaning. With the possible exception of one's occupation, in and of themselves all of the aforementioned things are emphatically insignificant when it comes to giving our lives enduring significance.

The bottom-line question is this: Am I basing my limited earthly time on the Fleeting Success (FS) factor—living for or amassing things, titles, and wealth—or am I basing my life on the Eternal Value (EV) factor—living as though how I've lived in this life will absolutely determine everything about my eternity?

To do proper justice to this most pressing question, we must take to heart that in eternity only what God deems significant will matter. It bears repeating that, unequivocally, any significance that we find in the brass of what the world considers important will not matter to God. In light of these certainties, we cannot compromise on the truths in God's Word if we expect our aggregate choices during our brief life to be counted significant in God's forever kingdom, or to meet His criteria for a life that has truly counted for His glory. Instead, we must take God at His Word and cultivate the mind-set that what will matter to Him *then* is what should matter to us *now*. If we desire true significance— wherein our earthly achievements last beyond this world—we must live with a backward orientation of time as we seek to fulfill God's purpose for our lives. Many of us tend to be extremely focused on things that are inconsequential compared to the final outcome of our earthly years. We would all do well to apply this Eternal Value mind-set to how we view and live our lives.

Leading a truly meaningful life is much like an open-book test. Although the questions are often difficult at times, we are confident that God has already given us clear guidelines for how to build eternally significant lives. If we continually seek His help and become very familiar with our textbook (the Bible), we can be assured that we'll get more answers right. Surely, how well we do on the open-book test will determine the results that we will receive on our final exam, when God judges how we've lived our earthly lives (see Ecclesiastes 12:14; Romans 2:6). But while this book posits that we must live ever mindful of the end of our temporal lives, I, nevertheless, want to emphasize that this does not preclude us from wholeheartedly embracing the journey. In fact, the very idea of living backward encompasses both the process *and* the end result.

THE DIVINE ART OF BUILDING

Speaking of process, I find it salient that Jesus was a carpenter. Although He is most assuredly our Bridegroom, our Savior, our Redeemer, our Lord, and indeed the King of the universe, could it be that He was a builder by trade to convey a higher spiritual truth about the building process, just as He did in so many of His teachings? Could it be that Jesus came to teach us the divine art of *building a life* that matters in God's forever kingdom? I want to share a profound story with you:

An elderly carpenter decided it was time to retire. Although the loss of income would be significant, he and his wife would nonetheless be able to get by. They'd sell their current house and get a smaller one with a lower mortgage payment. He informed his employer, a building contractor, of his plan. His boss was saddened to lose such a good worker. As a personal favor, he asked the carpenter if he would build just one more house before he retired. The carpenter agreed. But soon it became evident that his approach to the building project was anything but focused. Besides using inferior materials, he simply wasn't putting forth his best effort. In fact, his workmanship was plain shoddy.

After the carpenter finished the house, his employer inspected his work. Then he handed the carpenter the key to the house saying, "This house is yours—my gift to you."

This caught the carpenter completely off guard. And it left him devastated. If he had only known that he was building the house for himself, he would have done things very differently—he would have given his very best. Now he owned a house that was a far cry from the quality-built home that he could have and should have had.[4]

Our attitude toward life can be a lot like the carpenter's. We're easily distracted by the tyranny of the urgent or what's novel and exciting— e-mails, social media feeds, breaking news, hot new TV shows, and the

4. "The Carpenter's Story," Inspiration Peak, accessed October 10, 2014, http://www.inspirationpeak.com/cgi-bin/stories.cgi?record=22.

latest video games. Preoccupied with transient stuff and relatively trivial pursuits, we don't give enough importance to the monumental task
of building our very lives. Without a doubt, the busyness of life also
causes us to overlook or brush aside what really matters. Consequently,
we fail to redeem the time and to live on purpose.

We all know that with anything we do, we'll get out what we've put
in. Yet we neglect the fact that the final outcome of our lives is solely
determined by the way we've lived our days. Our tools and "building
materials" consist of how we invest the hours, money, resources, and
gifts God has given us, as well as the quality of the choices and decisions
that we make. If we're not intentional, we may come face-to-face with
the fact that we too could have done a better job. Or we may reflect on
the life we've built and realize that it does not accord with the life that
we really desired. Like the carpenter, we may find ourselves in the position of having to say, *If only I had known, I would have approached this
most critical building project with a far greater degree of seriousness. I
would have resolved to have built my life very differently.* This sort of
regret is the negative outcome of hindsight.

Each of us at one point or another has looked back on our lives or
on a particular situation and thought, *If only I knew back then what I
know now, my life would be different, or I wouldn't have made the same
choices.* At no other moment in your existence will this reality be more
profound than when you stand before God to give an account of your
life. Thankfully hindsight doesn't necessarily have to pertain to regret,
as it also enables us to draw upon what we've learned in the past to
make wiser future decisions. This is the wonderful or positive benefit
of hindsight, and we should certainly use it to our greatest advantage
as we go through life.

But there's an even better way, *a future-oriented way*, to view hindsight which truly turns it into a gift of time. It involves projecting to
your future eternal existence—to picture yourself looking back on the
sum total of your earthly years . . . and in that moment, discovering
that your reasons to rejoice and celebrate are far greater than those you

regret. Right now pause and reflect on this moment. As you look back on your time on earth, what kind of legacy or life story would you want to have created? The good news is that we can minimize the regret that we otherwise might have had. In contrast to the carpenter in the story above, each of us *can* still shape the final outcome of our lives. Now is the time to do just that! I assure you, you will want to have lived backward and leveraged to the fullest this gift of future-oriented hindsight.

BUILD WISELY

Starting now, think of yourself as building an eternal house. Each and every day the choices you make are like hammering a nail here, your decisions like laying a floor board there. Your actions are either erecting or tearing down walls. Indeed, your eternal future hinges on the quality of your workmanship and your steadfast commitment to the building project.

Take great care that you don't put forth shoddy effort. Build wisely instead, making God-honoring choices and decisions. Like a circle, your existence has no end. By living backward and capitalizing on the gift of hindsight, you can and will build a quality house that brings you great eternal joy, as well as God's glorious seal of approval.

Ultimately, we lead meaningful lives when our dreams, passions, and desires are rooted in the advancement of God's fame. As we honor God with our lives, He rejoices in and over us, and we bring great pleasure to His heart (see Isaiah 62:5; Zephaniah 3:17–18). But recall there's an exciting by-product: in delighting God's heart, He delights ours; in glorifying Him, our joy is fuller . . . more complete. Whether we're aware or not, this deep, soul-satisfying joy is what our thirsty hearts really yearn for; it is a joy far superior to the fleeting happiness we ultimately find in shallow, misdirected quests for significance.

Don't allow the transient pleasures and enticements of this world to cause you to lose your way; don't let them blind you to the incredible reality that to pursue God's glory is to also pursue your greatest ful-fillment. Think of me as your cheerleader, enthusiastically waving the pom-poms, urging you to be zealous for God's glory—the only glory that will last. With all my heart, I humbly pray that the wind of zeal will blow on these pages, causing them to rustle loudly with God's passion for His renown, and that the echoes you hear will bring encourage-ment and hope. However, I also pray that the contents of this book will challenge and convict hearts as we take inventory of our spiritual condition in the penetrating light of God's truth.

Indeed, we find true fulfillment as we wholly surrender our hearts to God. Scripture teaches, "For to me to live is Christ, and to die is gain" (Philippians 1:21). To live for Christ is gain, both temporal and eternal. However, we have to lose to win. Jesus plainly teaches, "If you try to hang on to your life, you will lose it. But if you give up your life for my sake, you will save it" (Matthew 16:25, New Living Translation). So I encourage you to gladly give or surrender the "brass" of worldly significance you may be desperately seeking but cannot keep in order to go for the gold and gain the eternal significance you can never, ever lose. After all, if you are God's, in a sense your "real" life begins when this temporal one ends. I'm certain you would want to have lived this fleeting life well. So would I!

Are you ready? Remember . . . time is precious. Life is short. Eternity is forever.

CHAPTER 2

YOU WANT TO MATTER

Desire that your life count for something great! Long
for your life to have eternal significance. Want this!
Don't coast through life without a passion.
—John Piper

Each of us is born with a deep longing. In order to live backward,
it's critical that we understand God's design for satisfying this innate
desire. Without this foundational knowledge, we'll all seek to gratify
this yearning through misguided pursuits that take us away from God's
path, causing us to forfeit a life of true significance.

WE LOVE THE CAMERA

It's 4:15 a.m. at 30 Rockefeller Plaza on Forty-Ninth Street in New York
City. The wind is whistling on this frigid winter night, but outside NBC's
Studio 1A, a small crowd of people has already gathered. Mission: Get
as close as possible to the studio's live broadcast area on the plaza. Goal:
Be seen on camera when the television network airs *The Today Show*
in less than five hours. But wait, isn't the temperature below freezing?

Why are these people here? Shouldn't they be fast asleep? If they are up this early, shouldn't they be doing something that really needs to be done, like laboring through the night and into the morning on a project deadline or getting ready for work? Call it fun, crazy, insane, whatever you'd like . . . these people are displaying zeal, although it may seem misdirected to some. If people have the zeal and determination to wait hours and hours in cold, miserable conditions just because they "need" to be seen on national TV, then just how strong is this drive or "need" to be known or to feel important?

WHERE EVERYBODY KNOWS YOUR NAME

I studied psychology in college and know this about the human psyche: we all want to matter. It's undeniable that each person desires to feel that they make a difference. This is also true for those who continually suppress this desire. We each want our lives to count—whether it's the savvy businesswoman who works eighteen-hour days in her quest for success; the missionary in a third-world country who makes tireless sacrifices to feed and educate the poor in order to make a difference; the young person who willingly takes ludicrous and unnecessary risks simply for the sake of applause; the Olympic athlete who subjects her body daily to the most grueling physical training in hopes of winning a gold medal; or the most indigenous person in the remotest place on earth seeking a place of honor in his tribe. Not a single person wants to feel insignificant. We want to achieve worthwhile goals; when we don't, we feel a deep sense of failure—perhaps the closest we come to being dead while our hearts are still beating. In fact, God Himself has hardwired this desire into each of us.

You may have heard of the highly rated TV show, *Cheers*, which aired between 1982 and 1993. Perhaps the reason for its huge success is captured in its theme song: "You want to go where everybody knows your name and they're always glad you came." There's much truth to this statement. We all want to belong and to feel accepted. This desire is the primary reason that we join various clubs and organizations. Deep down, each of us also longs to be "known." For example, I find it very meaningful whenever my husband does something he really dislikes— like several months ago when he helped me with desperately needed yard work—simply because he knows just how important it is to me. Recently, I felt very special when he took note of all the songs on one of my playlists and then surprised me by playing those same songs during a road trip.

In both situations, I experienced a deep sense of connectedness with my husband, as his actions conveyed not only his love for me but also his understanding of me. These tender expressions of his love also elicited a sudden spark, making my soul come alive and my heart swell with warm feelings toward him. Why? Because I felt "known"—my husband took into account what really matters to *me*, and in so doing, he uniquely affirmed me. Although it's intangible, there's something very powerful about this type of interconnectedness, which is why we all yearn to be intimately known. And this longing to be known—for who we are—is intrinsic to our desire to feel significant.

Of course, vice versa, the love sparks aren't set off when my husband acts in a way that is inconsistent with his intimate knowledge of me. Actually, it's far worse. I've discovered that even though it's unwitting, when my husband fails to acknowledge something that is of great importance to me, I suddenly feel somewhat emotionally disconnected from him. I've learned that if couples don't take care to address this disconnect right away, the emotional distance will only grow, negatively affecting all areas of their relationship. A failure to swiftly resolve an emotional disconnect helps explain why couples slowly drift apart and important relational needs go unmet; feeling disaffirmed where it matters most, intimacy begins to erode and relationships gradually lose their vibrancy.

On a different note, while technology has improved our lives, it is increasingly creating invisible walls that separate us from the human touch, voice, and experience. Not only does this separation undermine the sense of importance or significance that we should naturally derive from close relationships, but it also hinders our true connectedness with others. As a matter of fact, the explosive phenomenon of social networking is shedding light on the reality that we "live in an accelerating contradiction: the more connected we become, the lonelier we are."[5] Isolation gradually leads to loneliness. Far from affirming us, loneliness makes us miserable and depressed.

However, though it's great to be known and affirmed, it's important we understand two key truths. First, God our Creator ultimately designed us this way so that we could experience the deep joy of being intimately known by Him. Second, because God is the only one who completely knows us, *only* He can fully or perfectly satisfy our deep desire to be known. Our yearning to be known finds its end in God because His unending, unconditional fountain of love alone satisfies all of our restless desires. Indeed, it's in an intimate relationship with Him that we discover our greatest sense of belonging. Though it's not my intent to minimize hurts or suggest that we deny reality, when others inevitably fail to act in ways that affirm or acknowledge who we are, we can take heart in knowing that God our Father knows us intimately and perfectly—and He desires each of His children to experience a deepening awareness of this truth.

A POTENT DESIRE

The desire to feel significant is a potent force. We see this in the different twists and turns that we're willing to make in search of wealth, acceptance, commendation, and the like. For instance, in North America, the ubiquitous appeal of the American Dream heightens the desire for personal wealth and prestige. This drive, by the way, is deeply rooted in the notion of individualism woven into the fabric of

5.   Stephen Marche, "Is Facebook Making Us Lonely?" *Atlantic* (May 2012), 60–69.

this country's ideals. Consequently, we chase after success, searching for meaning wherever we believe it may be found. In addition to being overburdened by long work hours, many of us are bogged down by a smorgasbord of different activities such as additional schooling, chauffeuring children to a litany of activities, various hobbies, side business ventures, and a host of other commitments. Hectic schedules result in exhaustion and a state of burnout. Yet it's generally due to our own deliberate choices that we end up with little or no downtime or margin in our lives. The folly of this busyness is that it reinforces a mistaken sense of progress, which only exacerbates our overall dissatisfaction when we later discover just how little progress we've actually made.

I know this dynamic well. One of the side businesses that my husband and I were involved with early on in our marriage entailed his being away many weeknights and out of town most weekends presenting a business plan (often to complete strangers). Besides racking up thousands and thousands of miles on the family car in a relatively short period of time, we willingly chose to have him take precious time away from our young family because we desired financial freedom. Financial freedom to be able to give generously to worthwhile causes (which I later discovered can be a real snare), enjoy a lifestyle that afforded us the luxuries of life that we desired, and have the ability to work for ourselves. As I look back, we erroneously thought that financial freedom would instantly infuse our lives with a greater sense of meaning. We never did achieve any significant success with this venture, or with any of the other three businesses that we subsequently pursued. We reaped so little for all the time, money, and energy we had invested as well as the many sacrifices we had made. I now wonder what in the world were we thinking. Judging from the people I've seen and stories I've heard, we're not alone. We're eager to consider promising ventures that ultimately are disadvantageous or even worthless. At the end of the day, we somehow think they will enable us to find that elusive "something" which we believe will endow us with a greater sense of worth or value.

Respect. Wealth. Prestige. Applause. Recognition. Acclaim. The pursuit of these things is the primary reason many of us veer off God's path for our lives and subsequently lose our way.

I've discovered that the busyness of life is a master of deception. It hides under the radar, causing us to slowly and imperceptibly lose sight of what's most important, to the extent that we casually disregard the very purpose for which we live, move, and have our being: to delight the heart of God by bringing Him glory with our lives. Indeed, busyness is often an impostor of true success. I think we all know very busy people who have unwittingly sacrificed life's most precious gifts on the altar of success, leaving them with fractured marriages (or even divorce) or strained relationships with children, and sometimes both. The irony is that most do so firmly believing that they're making good and beneficial choices on behalf of their families.

Moreover, the desire for significance is so powerful that it affects our decisions and actions in ways we don't notice. Think for a moment about this universal tendency. People scream and go crazy, flail their arms in the air, smile, blush, or look away when they realize that their face has just flashed across the Jumbotron at a sporting event. Why? The simple answer is that they've been noticed. However brief it might have been, they momentarily felt important or seen. Hence, the greater the viewership audience, the more exaggerated the exuberance seems to be, as when people realize they're on national television with millions of viewers watching.

This is a very superficial illustration of our basic need to matter. Here are two more everyday examples:

Although largely unaware of this reality, a primary reason people are inclined to donate money to a cause is because the very act of giving or helping makes them feel significant. Sterling Stamos is an investment firm managing more than $3.5 billion. Each year, approximately 10 percent of the general partner's profits is allocated for social programs, primarily the advancement of global health. According to its president, Chris Stamos, "Philanthropy adds to staff morale and productivity, *gives clients a greater sense of fulfillment*, and increases the firm's financial capital through the appeal of good works"[6] (emphasis mine). Similarly, children and adults both tend to display negative behavior because they desperately want attention and figure that negative attention is actually better than none at all. For example, some students deliberately misbehave in order to attract teacher attention. These students don't care if the attention is to reprimand or praise. Both of these actions reveal the immense motivational power of the human drive for significance. People will do things that they otherwise might not do—both positive and negative—in order to feel important.

BURIED BUT ALIVE

As G. K. Chesterton aptly observed, "In everything on this earth that is worth doing, there is a stage when no one would do it except for necessity or honor."[7] How true! We understand that people are willing to endure difficult or extreme circumstances in order to meet a genuine need. Likewise, we admire people who willingly put themselves through incredibly harrowing hardships for the sake of honor.

But why would the folks outside the NBC studio willingly expose themselves to freezing temperatures—for several hours no less—merely to be seen on national television? Their actions seem to indicate that, in one sense, the desire for recognition may be a genuine need. It's not that people simply want to matter—people *desperately* want to matter. However, if this desire to matter is rooted in false beliefs about what we need, we'll likely become disillusioned with life. Therefore, we must allow the Holy Spirit, our Teacher and Helper, to guide us into what is true and pleasing to God (see John 14:26, 16:3; Romans 12:2). He searches our hearts and reveals our true needs, as well as the

6. Bill Clinton, *Giving: How Each of Us Can Change the World* (New York: Alfred A. Knopf, 2007), 23.

7. Cited in Elton Trueblood, *The Recovery of Family Life* (New York: Harper & Brothers, 1953), 50.

underlying motives or reasons behind what we want to pursue. As previously mentioned, God is zealous for us to purposefully live our lives for His glory and not our own. In our hearts, we are equally zealous for the sense of fulfillment this gives us. It is our God-given need.

Since you haven't laid this book down, I think it's fair to assume that you're taking serious stock of your life. Perhaps you realize that in the busyness of life, you've let some priorities slide, as I've done more times than I care to remember. For instance, there was a period in my life when I was too busy with my own agenda to regularly allocate time to study God's Word, which stunted my spiritual growth. During this same time, both my husband and I weren't intentional about setting aside time each day to teach God's Word to the three young children He had entrusted to us. Thankfully, God helped me to realign both of these priorities with His desires.

I also know just how easy it is to coast through life and to lose sight of the fact that focused effort must accompany our intrinsic desire to lead a purposeful life. Many people, for example, just talk about pursuing a certain goal but never become serious enough to actually do what it takes to achieve said goal. If you find that you've been overwhelmed with activity or coasting idly, choose this moment to reawaken yourself to the reality that, though latent—perhaps buried deep within the grooves of apathy or ruts of complacency that we tend to imperceptibly create over the years—you, nevertheless, still desire to lead a meaningful life. This is to say, although our primal yearning to truly matter is often smothered by the pressures and demands of life, it is nevertheless alive and well.

This is why the desire to lead a life of significance sometimes arises when we least expect it, as when we watch, say, a documentary, and it unexpectedly awakens something deep within us. Generally, when we find our hearts are stirred by this potent desire (provided we're not seeking to advance our selfish ambitions or embrace the things of this world), it serves to enlighten us to the raw materials of deep needs and passions that God Himself has planted in us. Things such as cruelty, hypocrisy, injustice, and discrimination which elicit anger, empathy, resistance, or deep hatred in us or rouse us into action likewise provide clues: they reveal how God has hardwired us to be a catalyst for redemptive change in the world.

The following sections have examples intended to highlight our instinctive desire to feel significant. However, they just might hint at how much we imperceptibly lose sight of what really matters, even the simple joys of everyday life. It's all too easy to forget to cherish each day: to gratefully rejoice in the goodness of God dancing all around us; to invest in building God's kingdom on the earth; and to appreciate and spend time with our loved ones, especially our spouses and children.

I don't know where life finds you today, but wherever you find yourself, it's time to face two facts: First, our situations are primarily a result of the aggregate choices and decisions we ourselves have made. Second, although we may have experienced extremely difficult circumstances that were entirely beyond our control, how we've chosen to respond to them has greatly affected how our lives have turned out so far, for better or worse. It's not my intent to minimize any trials or challenges you may have experienced; I'm simply saying that the extent to which we allow God to shape us in the midst of life's trials carries great weight.

No matter the feelings these examples elicit, with God on our side, there's thankfully always the promise of a brighter tomorrow. We can always make a fresh start and begin to reprioritize our lives. Recognizing that time waits for no one, we can choose each and every day to live life with intention. Indeed, any day is a great day to begin cultivating the seeds of our God-ordained purpose. Properly nurtured, these seeds or God-given desires have the potential to bring forth the harvest of a life richly fulfilled in Christ. Psalm 37:4 teaches, "Delight yourself in the Lord and he will give you the desires of your heart." Therefore, it's important to emphasize that to relinquish our self-centered desires in favor of God's desires for us doesn't mean that we don't get to do something meaningful or that we necessarily have to abandon something that we love. Not at all. That's because God's desires for our lives are far, far better than any desires that He may call us to surrender. Even if you dreamed up the most wonderful plan for your life, God's thoughts and intents for you—*both now and forever*—are far, far greater than anything you could even begin to imagine.

A WIFE WORTH HER WEIGHT IN GOLD

Have you ever read an acknowledgment in a book where the author says something along these lines:

> I am very thankful for my wonderful wife of twenty years who is so beautiful—from the inside out—that she makes me the happiest man on the planet. She has brought out and continues to bring out the very best in me. Year after sweet year she patiently and lovingly continues to help me become a better man, husband, and father! Her kindness, steadfast love, and deep devotion have beautifully adorned our marriage . . . always.

Clearly, this is a man, who, if sincere, truly loves, admires, cherishes, and appreciates his wife. This word of thanks is the stuff romantic movie scripts are made from. If you're a married man reading such an acknowledgment, you might beam and think, *Wow, his wife sounds just like mine!* or *I sure wish I could say that about my wife.* At any rate, you'd find yourself subconsciously comparing your wife to the author's. You may also wonder whether you've "pulled your weight" to create the kind of nurturing marriage that would motivate your wife to treat you in the same way. If by all indications you have, you'd likely experience what I'll call a "yes, I'm the man" fist-pump moment. I'm guessing that for the typical guy—who thinks in black and white—this (hopefully humble) macho display would aptly capture your instinctive desire to be validated as a terrific husband. However, you'd most likely be quite dismayed if you recognized that over the years you could have done more to stoke the flames of your marriage.

Let's switch gears. What sort of emotions would reading the words of this acknowledgment invoke in you if you were a married woman? It's quite likely your mind might drift away from the book, momentarily distracted by whether you too matter like this to your own husband. I admit that's what I'd do. You also might instantaneously begin to wonder whether your husband, if given the same opportunity, would say something that tender about you. Perhaps you might brim with confidence that he would or has even done so in the past. Such positive thoughts would affirm you as a wife and give you a renewed sense of satisfaction regarding your marriage.

But what if, on the other hand, you surmised that, as far as you could tell, your husband most likely wouldn't say something that commendable about you? This would sting, leaving you feeling hurt and sad or maybe even depressed. Far from affirming you, it would break your heart. The point I'm making is that if you're a wife, your mind would instinctively go down one of two thought paths. This is true for the simple reason that you harbor a deep desire to be treasured like the wife described in the above acknowledgment. And this desire is an expression of your innate longing for significance as a wife who is appreciated, loved, and adored.

STOPPING TO SMELL THE ROSES . . .

Imagine you're a young father listening as one of your buddies vividly describes his joy in having become a new dad. Your attention is arrested when he mentions that he sat for more than ninety minutes gazing at his newborn daughter as she slept. Amazed, you think, *Wow! Did he just say he spent more than an hour just watching his baby sleep?* Sparing no details as he gushes out blow by blow how he took in the beauty and sheer wonder of this precious new life, you can't help but notice how he spontaneously used all his senses to describe the experience: how he gazed into her big brown eyes, listened to her softly breathing, kissed the curves of her little face, gently stroked her tiny fingers and toes, and deeply inhaled the fragrance of her petal-soft skin. *OK*, you think, *enough already . . . I get the picture!* The dagger comes when he adds that he did nothing else but just sit there—no TV, no cell phone, no iPad—completely captivated by his sweet bundle of joy.

Suddenly, his voice has trailed off and you're no longer listening. Distracted, you find yourself thinking back to when your now three-year-old daughter was born. You try to remember the details but soon realize there's so much you've already forgotten. Nevertheless, you know for certain that somehow, it never once occurred to you to slow down, turn off the noise of life, stop everything else you were doing, and just "take in" your baby as this new dad has done. It slowly dawns on you that the missed opportunities to just revel in the precious gift of your newborn daughter is a microcosm of the many priceless moments you've allowed to slip through your fingers like sand. Overcome by regret, you might resolve to do a better job of stopping to smell the roses.

This isn't the only response, though. The other possible scenario is that you clearly remember how your daughter was as an infant because you indeed spent time—plenty of time—with her. You instantly recall how a smile lit up her face the moment you entered her room to get her from her crib; you remember how she smelled just after her evening bath; and you can still hear her delightful squeal whenever you scooped her up and nestled her in your arms for her favorite activity—to hear Daddy read another silly bedtime story. A nostalgic joy washes over you as you reflect on the web of happiness that this darling child has tenderly woven around your heart.

At any rate, your friend's exuberant sharing of this tender time with his daughter would likely have prompted you to ponder how good a dad you've been. Why? Because regardless of how much or how little you've invested in your child's life up to this point, you naturally desire to experience the satisfaction that comes from being a great dad. You want to have a deep-down assurance that besides fulfilling your responsibility to put a roof over your daughter's head, food on the table, and clothes on her back, you're also treasuring priceless moments with her. In short, you long to measure up as a wonderful dad, and if you do, you derive a deep sense of value and significance. By the way, if you're a parent, I'd like to share this salient quote: "If you want to be in your child's memories *tomorrow*, you have to be in his or her life *today*!"[8] Don't let the years slip through your hands.

I DID IT MY WAY!

Without a doubt, God desires us to experience a sense of significance from our varied roles in life, be it a mother, husband, wife, secretary, Sunday school teacher, student-athlete, pastor, teacher, or youth leader. Because He instituted them, God also cares a great deal about marriages and families. Thus, the instinctive desires mentioned in the examples above are all good and healthy desires to cultivate and pursue. Of course, there are many such examples, but each requires an investment of time and effort in order to achieve meaningful results. Although a great many of us entertain dreams of one day changing the world, allowing God to use us as His redemptive instruments in the transformation of our homes and families is one of the pivotal ways to lead a life of significance and influence the world for Christ.

Even when pursuing healthy desires, we must be careful to keep them in their proper places; otherwise, they can very easily become idols. An idol may be simply defined as anything we focus our time, talents, attention, and financial resources on to the extent that it undermines or jeopardizes our relationship with God. It is anything or anyone that usurps the preeminence that God alone deserves to have in

---

8.   As quoted by Barbara Johnson.

our hearts and lives. People idolize everything from their children to their hobbies, their Facebook accounts to their careers, and everything in between. The list is seemingly endless. Obsessed with their physical features, some people, in a sense, even idolize themselves. Moreover, there are times when even a well-meaning desire, such as staying physically fit, eventually morphs into an idol. Although God commands us to have no other gods before Him, we are naturally hardheaded and stubborn (see Exodus 34:9). This reality is plainly taught in Isaiah 53:6: "We all, like sheep, have gone astray, each of us has turned to his own way."

Left to ourselves, each and every one of us has a proclivity to rebel against God; we naturally transgress or go against His desire for our lives. At times, we try to manipulate God in our attempts to receive His gifts and blessings. In our stubbornness and arrogance, we forget that God Almighty stooped down and entered the world He created in order to save us from the wrath and condemnation that our sins justly deserved. Therefore, when we live for ourselves, we act as though we are our own masters, or that God should serve us. Our attitude is reminiscent of the dog that walks out onto the front porch, looks up and sees the moon in the night sky, and then barks at the moon, as if believing that his barking prowess is the reason that the moon exists. Similarly, it's easy for us to go through life believing and acting as though we can live on our own terms and will later triumphantly proclaim, "I did it my way!" We mistakenly believe that we can find true contentment in this life apart from God. This is all wrong! Since Adam and Eve, humans have been trying to find fulfillment in something apart from God. In fact, all of history is "the long terrible story of man trying to find something other than God which will make him happy."[9]

There's an African folk tale about how the spider ended up with a small waist. It goes like this: Spider is conflicted. He's been invited to a feast and to a dinner party—on opposite sides of the river. Besides thinking himself clever, Spider also happens to be very greedy. So he

9.   C. S. Lewis, *Mere Christianity* (New York: HarperCollins, 2003), 49.

hatches what he believes is an ingenious plan. He ties a rope around his waist and instructs the people on one side of the river to tug on it when it's time to eat. He takes the other end of the rope and gives it to the folks on the other side of the river with the exact same instructions. As it turns out, dinner was held at the same time on both sides of the river.

We are all a lot like Spider. While we're familiar with the maxim, "You can't have your cake and eat it too," we naturally want to eat the cake of the world (which is contrary to God's desires) and yet also have God on our side. Because we choose to follow our self-will, we audaciously believe that we actually can achieve this impossibility. Such thinking is terribly misguided. To live for the fleeting things of this world is ultimately sheer folly. First of all, after we have taken our final breath, absolutely nothing in this temporal world will still be ours; secondly, we risk incurring the gravest consequence of all—potentially not joining God in the life hereafter.

Moreover, the Bible clearly teaches that we will face one of two certain realities after we pass from this earthly life. We will either spend eternity in Heaven, a glorious place of unspeakable joy, or we will spend eternity in Hell, a place of unimaginable torment and suffering. Our eternal (and conscious) destiny, then, is one of either everlasting joy or everlasting suffering (see Matthew 13:41–42, 25:46; Mark 9:43–44). "Having the cake of this world" unequivocally will not be an option: we will either have God or we will have absolutely nothing. Actually, the latter state will be far worse than having nothing—no mind can possibly conceive what it will be like to be utterly separated from any hint of God's grace and goodness. It is essential, then, that we humble ourselves before the One who holds our eternal destiny in His hands.

LOST IN NEW YORK CITY

Charles Spurgeon, a minister during the 1800s, saliently noted, "Where God is unacknowledged, the mind is void of judgment. Where God is not worshiped, the heart of man becomes a ruin."[10] Therefore, if we want to get our lives right, it follows that we must first get right with God. Our communion with God is by far the most paramount relationship we can have. Needless to say, this will require investment of our time and energy. However, there is absolutely nothing of greater importance in our lives than seeking to know the God of the universe who created us and calls us His own. What He has revealed of Himself transcends all other knowledge or wisdom that we could ever seek. As J. I. Packer aptly states, "The highest science, the loftiest speculation, the mightiest philosophy, which can ever engage the attention of a child of God, is the name, the nature, the person, the work, the doings, and the existence of the great God, whom He calls his Father . . . For nothing will so enlarge the intellect, nothing so magnify the whole soul of man, as a devout, earnest, continued investigation of the great subject of the deity."[11] To this, I can only add my resounding "Amen!"

It truly cannot be overstated that seeking to know God is of the utmost importance in life. To adopt an example used by Packer, just as it would be cruel to take someone from a remote village in Africa or Asia and plop him down in the middle of New York City, leaving him to completely fend for himself, "so we are cruel to ourselves if we try to live in this world without knowing about the God whose world it is and who runs it."[12] On the contrary, those who purposefully apply themselves to knowing God become more and more convinced that He is infinitely worthy of their zealous pursuit. Captivated by His awesomeness and unparalleled beauty, they are never satisfied with their current experience of God and long for still more of Him—richer communion, deeper intimacy, and a greater awareness of His indwelling presence and power. Their very lives become a song of worship, punctuated by a refrain that epitomizes surrender to their King: Lord, above

....

10. Charles Spurgeon, *The Fullness of Joy* (New Kensington: Whitaker House, 1997), 21.

11. J. I. Packer, *Knowing God* (Downer's Grove: InterVarsity Press, 1973), 17.

12. Ibid., 19.

all, may You be pleased! And like clocks, they set their hearts to beat
for Him alone . . . to live for Him alone.

YOUR INVITATION

Many of us have bought into the false notion that this kind of personal
fellowship with God is reserved for only some of His children. Not
true! God invites you, me, and each of His children to enjoy daily,
intimate fellowship with Him. For a multitude of reasons, the richness
of individual experiences will vary by degrees, but it is God's desire
that each of His children earnestly say of Him: "My flesh and my heart
may fail: but God is the strength of my heart, and my portion forever,"
"I am your shield; your reward shall be very great," and "Worthy are
you, our Lord and God, to receive glory and honor and power" (Psalm
73:26; Genesis 15:1; Revelations 4:11). This heart posture delights the
heart of God. This is what truly matters! When we pursue God's divine
design for our lives to bring Him pleasure, there will not be an inkling
of regret.

FANNING THE DESIRE

So are you now more resolved and determined to live out God's eternal
purpose for your life? I pray you are. I sincerely hope you're beginning
to sense a stirring in your heart for your life to count for nothing less
than God's glory. No doubt, as the Bible cannot lie: "Whoever finds
his life will lose it, and whoever loses his life for my sake will find it"
(Matthew 10:39; see also Matthew 16:25; Luke 9:24). I want to both
encourage and exhort you to lose your life so that what you choose
to do and become in this fleeting breath of time will count in God's
eternal kingdom!

More than you could possibly fathom, God Himself is very passionate for your life to matter! The question is: Are you? Do you sincerely want to build the edifice of a truly significant life? If so, then embrace the gift of hindsight and live backward, pursuing a life lived for God's glory. Fan the flames of your desire by diving in—with all your heart, mind, soul, and strength! God is trustworthy, and His promises ensure that you will not regret the decision to follow him for all eternity. In fact, the rewards for relentlessly pursuing God are staggering and quite literally out of this world: "no eye has seen, nor ear heard, nor the heart of man imagined, what God has prepared for those who love him" (1 Corinthians 2:9).

YOUR WILLINGNESS IS KEY

I mentioned earlier that this book is your road map to pursue and reclaim what matters most in this life. But you must first be willing to be led. God primarily leads and guides us by His Spirit and by His Word, which is "a lamp to my feet and a light to my path" (Psalm 119:105), even during the darkest times of our lives. His Word illumines and renews our minds, teaching us to have an undivided heart—to forsake ourselves and give up the right to do as we please. Led by His Spirit, we learn to walk in the paths of truth and be devoted to God by turning away from anything that would hinder our relationship with Him. And we increasingly desire to follow the route laid out by the divine GPS even when it doesn't make one iota of sense.

But as you'll recall, we are all like sheep that have gone astray; we're so easily tempted to wander from the fold. If we are to honor the Lord with our lives, we desperately need to be near our Shepherd's staff. A line from a well-known hymn, "Where He Leads Me," states, "Where He leads me I will follow." If you are ready to be led so that your life will forever count for God and His kingdom, I encourage you to bear these words of the late Elisabeth Elliot in mind:

Experience has taught me that [Jesus] the [Good] Shepherd is far more willing to show His sheep the path than the sheep are to follow. He is endlessly merciful, patient, tender, and loving. If we, His [clueless] and wayward sheep, really want to be led, we will without fail be led. Of that I am sure.[13]

Baa, baa, baa, I stand in full and joyous agreement!

Suffice to say, you are not a mistake or an accident. In a world where many forces may have seemingly conspired to make you feel unseen, insignificant, and unimportant, you do matter to God! You exist for a specific, God-ordained purpose! Indeed, there's a vacuum deep inside of you that can only be filled as you ful*fill* God's particular purpose for your life. The time for you to fulfill your purpose or be prepared for it is now. Throughout life's ebbs and flows, joys and sorrows, highs and lows—in dependence on God—do all within you to wisely redeem the time. Our life clocks are ticking, persistently counting down the time we each have left to make this vapor of life count.

Get ready, get set, and let's get started . . . *together!*

---

13. Elisabeth Elliot, *Keep a Quiet Heart* (Grand Rapids: Revell, 2008), 155.

CHAPTER 3

....

PERFECTLY FASHIONED FOR THE GRAND STAGE OF LIFE

> To live is the rarest thing in the world. Most
> people exist, that is all.
> —Oscar Wilde

In this chapter, we'll explore our immeasurable worth to God—why He made us and how He sees us—and look at the ramifications of His purpose in uniquely fashioning each of us for the display of His glory. A solid understanding of these truths is vital to living backward.

MOUNTAINTOP EXPERIENCES

But first a word of caution, especially if you're someone like me who can't seem to get enough of reading and studying about God in a desire to draw ever closer to Him. I used to read about the exciting or intriguing "mountaintop experiences" with God that godly men and women had, and I desired—at times unwittingly coveted—a similar experience for myself. As I matured, though, I realized this desire was neither scriptural nor honoring to God, but I'm not alone in the confusion I felt.

While it's certainly fine to admire fellow brothers and sisters in Christ, it is wrong to desire the same experiences or circumstances that God has allowed another person to walk through. Although this misguided desire may not seem all that harmful, it has the potential to derail a person's faith walk. First, because God draws each person to Himself in a different way. Second, many folks (including Bible teachers, evangelists, pastors, authors) rely on their personal experiences to establish or validate a biblical principle or truth. It should be the other way around. Biblical truths are valid simply because they are biblical. Any encounter with God should allow the heart to see the person, nature, or work of Christ; but if an experience is void of a biblically accurate revelation of Christ, it is not a revelation from God—and it can lead others astray.

I was misled earlier in my walk by false teachings that included this inaccuracy, and we live in a time when New Age beliefs, humanistic ideas, and Eastern mysticism are increasingly infiltrating the evangelical church. So Christians need to stand vigilantly for the purity of the gospel.

As we seek to experience God, we must always remember that any encounters we have with the Lord are ours and not someone else's. Hence, each of us must be careful to never draw a general conclusion about what God is doing in our personal lives and then bring it to bear on someone else's life. There may be a natural tendency to think that just because God is dealing with you about a particular sin, that your best friend, husband, mother, sister should also confront the same sin in his or her life. In contrast to a true biblical judgment, this attitude involves subjectively evaluating others (which Matthew 7:1 warns against) and trying to fix them based on our own standards. It is an attempt to play the divine role of the Holy Spirit in the lives of others.

However, the Spirit of God does not need or welcome our help. Not at any time. Only He knows what each of us needs as we all are works in progress. We are each at distinct places in the sanctifying process of living as the transformed people God has called us to be.

Although it's also very tempting to evaluate our spiritual growth by comparing ourselves to others, Jesus is the only standard by which we must measure our progress. His perfect example of holiness alone is what we must imitate or pattern our lives after (see 1 Peter 2:21).

Oswald Chambers sums up well the idea of letting God be God in the lives of others: "Never make a principle out of your experience; let God be as original with other people as He is with you."[14] God's wooing, drawing, and eventual love relationship with each of His children will look starkly different from one to the next. Indeed it should.

SNOWFLAKES . . . NO TWO ARE THE SAME!

To begin to see our relationship with God the way He sees it, we must see ourselves the way He sees us. Consider for a moment that no two snowflakes have ever been alike, ever! Think of all the inches, feet, layers, and mountains of snow that have ever fallen in various parts of the world. Now, try to mentally combine these incredible treasuries of snow. I don't know about you, but that is more snow than I can possibly begin to imagine. Yet it's a marvel to think that when viewed under a microscope, each snowflake has a unique, intricate design.

Scripture teaches us not to worry about anything. In Matthew 6:28–34, God assures us that if He can make the lilies of the field grow and clothe them in splendor without any effort on their part, how much more can He also buttress His children and provide them with everything they need. Similarly, does God not value those whom He has created *in His own image* immeasurably more than He does snowflakes? And if He has the divine wisdom and creativity to be so original with snow so that no two crystals (composed of only hydrogen and oxygen molecules, mind you) are ever alike, how much more creativity is at God's divine disposal when we factor in the intangible characteristics

....

14. Oswald Chambers, *My Utmost for His Highest* (Uhrichsville: Barbour Publishing, Inc., 1963), June 13 entry.

such as personality, temperament, and unique gifts and talents? Then over all this, add the complexities of genetics and cultural influences. When we view our lives in this way, it's easy to see how each of us is truly God's unique masterpiece. I like how Dr. Seuss, the famous children's author, simply puts it, "Today you are you that is truer than true. There is no one alive who is youer than you."

GOD'S KINGDOM COMPANY

If we were to think of God as an auto manufacturer, then each of us is a special make and model in His Kingdom Company. Take the Honda auto company, for example. It makes vehicles for several purposes. Some are used as crash cars to enhance safety performance, while others are demo cars used for test-driving. The overwhelming majority of cars are manufactured for consumer purchase. Moreover, Honda reserves the express right to decide what the make, model, and color (both interior and exterior) of each car will be, what features it will have, and whether it ends up on a showroom floor. Ultimately, each car is manufactured with predetermined specifications and for a designated purpose.

It is not much different with God and His creatures, though our purpose is far more sophisticated and wonderful than that of a car's could ever be! (And God doesn't use anyone as a test dummy!) Not only has God uniquely created us, He has also equipped each of us for a special role or designated purpose. If, like me, you are awed that no two snowflakes are ever alike, how much more should we marvel and rejoice that God has an incredibly beautiful plan for each of our lives, one so highly individualized that no other person was designed to fulfill it. As such, the most fundamental way that we glorify God is to wholly embrace our unique gifts and abilities and then intentionally pursue His specific plan for our lives. When we do—when we connect with our God-given purpose—we experience our greatest fulfillment, affirming that our greatest joy and God's renown are interwoven.

To take the manufacturing concept one step further, when the Honda Accord wins an award, to whom does the credit go? Will it be the automaker or the actual test car that was driven? Of course, the Honda Motor Company will receive all the acclaim, accolades, and recognition. The same should be true of us with regards to God, our Maker. God alone is the source of everything that we have, down to the very breath in our lungs; without Him we can do absolutely nothing.

Therefore, for anything noteworthy that we accomplish or any praise and admiration that we receive, God alone should receive all the glory. Just like the Accord should never boast about itself (if it could), we should be careful to humbly deflect all the praise and attention from ourselves to God. Yet due to our prideful hearts, the natural tendency is to think of ourselves less as the Accord and more like the Honda Motor Company, acting as though we designed and made ourselves, are great in and of ourselves, and have accomplished success in our own strength. To do so is to essentially rob God of the credit that is rightfully His. Conversely, God is well pleased when we acknowledge His handiwork in our lives, giving Him all of the glory for the special gifts He has deposited in us as well as anything good that comes out of us.

PERFECTLY FASHIONED

You might think that we should instinctively know and embrace our God-given uniqueness. However, from a very early age we are conditioned to desire to be more like someone else. It seems almost unavoidable. If you've ever observed little boys, for example, you'll often find them pretending to be their favorite superhero. It's just the way that they play. The media plays a significant role in our conditioning. It constantly bombards us with information, influencing us to act a certain way or be like someone else. In fact, much of what we see and hear—slogans, billboards, commercials, TV shows, movies, and a host of other stimuli—reinforces this notion.

For instance, do you remember the extremely popular "Be Like Mike" Gatorade commercial from the summer of 1991? The ads highlighted some of the amazing athletic feats of Michael Jordan, arguably one of the greatest players to have ever played the game of basketball. The ad campaign was primarily intended to persuade people to drink Gatorade. Part of the catchy jingle goes like this, "Sometimes I dream that he is me; you've got to see that's how I dream to be . . . If I could be like Mike, like Mike, oh, if I could be like Mike, be like Mike, be like Mike, be like Mike." I can't help but wonder how many boys and young men got caught up in the hype of the commercial and, rather than pursuing an understanding of their unique gifts, wanted to become just like Jordan instead of who they'd been created to be. As recently as February 2015, Gatorade capitalized on the overwhelming success of the "Be Like Mike" ad by releasing a digitally remastered version. Now an entirely new generation of young people will be dazzled to subscribe to the mistaken goal espoused by this and other similar commercials.

If we're honest with ourselves, we'll admit that even when we've matured into adults, we can harbor a secret desire to be more like someone else. For example, we might wish we had someone else's hair texture, desire another person's physique, or covet someone's oratory skills or leadership ability. Yet we each have the eye and skin color, hair type, body shape, height, temperament, personality, and strengths that God specifically wanted us to have. When we truly grasp this truth, we won't ever again question the unique physical characteristics and innate gifts that God has given to us.

But what if you have to deal with something that has implications far greater than, say, mere height? What if you were born, for example, with a congenital heart condition or are afflicted with a mental or physical handicap that severely limits what you are capable of doing? I don't want to in any way make light of your specific challenge. But I do want to reassure you that although such circumstances are painful and very difficult to accept, in God's mysterious providence, they too are part of His unique plan and purpose for your life. I encourage you to read Psalm 139 in its entirety. It paints a vivid description of the great care God took in creating each person, intricately and beautifully fashioning each of us in our mother's womb. The critical and practical application of these truths is that God can accomplish in each of us whatever He desires, both despite and in spite of the limitations and circumstances that we face.

As a matter of fact, Scripture itself is replete with story after story which underscore that God is more than able to take our handicaps, disappointments, disabilities, weaknesses, shortcomings, insecurities, and, indeed, everything about us, including our past—sins, shame, failures, scars, and disappointments—and use them to showcase His glory. (We'll look at a few examples later in this chapter.) Nothing about your physical makeup or life experience is a mistake or outside of God's sovereign control.

Although it's counterintuitive to us, God actually does some of His best work in the most difficult of circumstances. I learned this first-hand. As a young adult, I eagerly looked forward to being a wife and then a mother. After two years of marriage, I was elated to discover that I was pregnant. Well into my second trimester, I all of a sudden started to have labor pains. As my husband drove me to the emergency room, I was very hopeful that my doctor would be able to help me continue the pregnancy. But his evaluation left me devastated. I learned that I was carrying not one but two babies, and one had already entered the birth canal much too early. There was nothing my doctor could do to reverse the situation. On that fateful November day, I gave birth to a daughter, and, on the following day, a son, but neither survived.

Fast-forward a year later when I found out I was pregnant again. You can imagine my joy and elation when I learned that I was again carrying another set of twins. At the end of my first trimester, my doctor performed a procedure to help ensure that I would not go into early labor as before. Everything went well. Bed rest was prescribed for the remainder of my pregnancy, and I felt like a mother hen happily sitting on her eggs to keep them warm. I wish I could say this story had a happy ending. But it didn't. In the middle of the night and without any warning, my amniotic sac ruptured. As I stood in the shower, the life-giving fluid trickling out of me, I instinctively knew that my babies' survival was grim, as I was only twenty-three weeks along. I immediately began to pray, begging and pleading with God to please save my precious babies. After being admitted to the hospital, I was placed on the delivery floor, surrounded by fetal heart monitors and sounds of life as other babies took their first breath. But God didn't say yes to my prayer. I felt cruelly out of place as I waited to naturally give birth to babies whose hearts had already stopped beating.

Both losses were devastating. They left me perplexed, as I had three sisters who all had experienced several smooth pregnancies and deliveries. Yet in my grief and utter sadness, God empowered me to open and entrust my heart to Him. Then something amazing happened. I can't quite explain how He did it, but somehow God gave me the ability to accept that what had happened was part of His unique plan for my life, even though I was as yet relatively young in my spiritual growth. I guess you can call it the faith of resignation, because as I grieved the loss of these precious babies, crying myself to sleep night after night, I never felt angry at God or questioned, "Why me?" Instead, God used these pregnancy losses to help me keenly grasp that in my youthful zeal I was not in control of how everything in my life unfolded; He was. God was indeed doing a great work in me because, without this understanding, I wouldn't have recognized the absolute necessity as His child to relinquish all my dreams and desires to Him.

In the midst of both losses, God used my recognition of His sovereignty over all He created to draw me closer to Him and to strengthen my ability to not only trust Him more fully with my life but also trust in His good plans for my life. Scripture assured me that "The Lord is close to the brokenhearted; he rescues those whose spirits are crushed

(Psalm 34:18, New Living Translation). God's Word is true! Through prayer, the study of the Bible, and the writing of poetry (that drew upon His many promises), I experienced God's comfort, peace, and strength. I'm keenly aware that this isn't everyone else's story of pregnancy loss. I'm also not suggesting that being angry with God or questioning Him are not a normal part of the grieving process for many. I'm simply sharing how God worked in my life and how the faith He supernaturally instilled in me shielded me from losing hope and feeling defeated during those difficult times.

Following the subsequent joyous births of two healthy sons, I experienced yet another pregnancy loss. This time, a stillbirth in my eighth month. I'll never forget the anguish of kissing the perfectly formed face of a longed-for daughter. God, it seemed, had given me yet another opportunity to completely yield to His sovereign orchestration of my life. Amid bitter disappointment and heart-wrenching pain, He was again faithful. In my weakness and despair, God was indeed strong (see 2 Corinthians 12:9). He tenderly reminded me that He was in control. Just as He had blessed me with two sons after my previous miscarriages, I could trust in His special plans for my life.

Since I had grown in my faith after the previous pregnancy losses, I then desired to testify about God's goodness and faithfulness, not just humbly accept my plight. I wanted to walk out the reality that, no matter what, by faith followers of Christ can and must trust God when we walk through painful and extremely difficult circumstances. I clung to God's promise that "Hope deferred makes the heart sick, but a desire fulfilled is a tree of life" (Proverbs 13:12). Amazingly, exactly one year to the day after I experienced the stillbirth, I discovered that the baby I was carrying was another girl. Three months later, joy erupted like a volcano in my heart when I give birth to a healthy daughter. I've since taken to heart the scriptural teaching: "And we know that God causes everything to work together for the good of those who love God and are called according to his purpose for them" (Romans 8:28, New Living Translation). Scripture also teaches, "The Lord is righteous in all his ways and kind in all his works" (Psalm 145:17). Indeed God does *all* things—not some things—marvelously well (see Psalms 116:7, 139:14). Then and now, I continue to cling to the blessed hope that some glorious day God has promised to "wipe every tear from [our] eyes" (Revelations 21:4). May our Father use the precious truths in His Word to continually reassure us and deepen our trust in His divine perfections, especially in those incredibly hard realities that we greatly struggle to grasp or understand.

DOES THE CLAY QUESTION THE POTTER?

Even though I realize that the following statement may sound rather simple or obvious, I believe it still needs to be stated: it is neither spiritually healthy nor beneficial to desire to be anyone other than who God made you to be or to wish that God would work in you exactly as He has in another person. At best, such thinking breeds frustration, and, at worst, it dishonors God. In fact, to not embrace *all* of who we are or to desire to be different than how God has made us deeply grieves the heart of God. Isaiah 43:6–7 states, "bring my sons from afar and my daughters from the end of the earth, everyone who is called by my name, whom I created for my glory, whom *I formed and made*" (emphasis mine). Did you catch that? Though we may not be aware, our tendency to want to be other than whom God has made us actually calls into question God's wisdom in fashioning us.

To doubt His perfect handiwork in our lives, however subtly, also carries the implication that God somehow made a mistake when He designed us or apportioned our unique gifts. God revealed this truth to me once when I was questioning an aspect of my physical makeup. I was born with clubbed feet. Well over eighteen months old, I was still not walking. Through a string of miraculous interventions, a German orthopedist aboard a traveling hospital ship made it all the way to the west coast of Africa and performed the needed surgery that hitherto had been unavailable to correct my feet. From the ages of five through twelve, I was pigeon-toed and had to wear special orthopedic shoes that were very unattractive, to say the least. I remember being extremely self-conscious of my feet and how I walked. As an adult, certain types of shoes looked fine on me, but most didn't. At times, I resented the fact that I couldn't just purchase a pair of shoes that I liked and that fitted because they didn't look attractive on my feet. Even when I found a pair that did, they wound up hurting my feet each time I wore them. During those times when I complained about my feet, I had no idea that my resentment was indirectly calling into question how God had chosen to make me.

Then one day I read Psalm 139 and became overwhelmed by its beautiful imagery capturing just how wondrously God had formed me and knitted me together in my mother's womb. It was then I fully grasped that for some reason God, in His infinite wisdom, had allowed me to be born with clubbed feet. In addition, I was in a breech position (feetfirst rather than headfirst entering the birth canal) when it came time for my mother to give birth. Just minutes before the doctors were about to perform a caesarean section, God did something incredulous: although full-term, I suddenly turned and my mother had me naturally. I've always known this fact about my birth. However, this Psalm solidified my grasp of God's intervention in my life even before I was born. It also helped me to understand that it had been God's divine prerogative whether my feet had been corrected and that, either way, He was still God and He was still good. I'm indeed ever grateful that my heavenly Father chose to correct my feet for the display of His glory in my life, especially given the sad reality that I've seen both children and adults born in the great United States whose clubbed feet have not been corrected. This sobering recognition deepened my trust not only in God's unique plans for each of His children but also in His providential and fatherly care as well.

Yet I realize that for many it's often hard not to blame God for the trials, tragedies, setbacks, disappointments, and hardships in life. At times, even devout Christians unapologetically distrust God. Life has dealt them an "unfair" blow, and it seems God has either ignored them or hasn't done anything about it. I really think many of us simply don't realize that questioning God's workings in our lives betrays our innate human tendency to think big thoughts of ourselves and small thoughts of our all-wise Creator and Maker. Isaiah 45:9 explicitly admonishes us not to have such an attitude: "Woe to him who strives with him who formed him, a pot among earthen pots! Does the clay say to him who forms it, 'What are you making?' or 'Your work has no handles'?"

Though it may be hard to embrace, the Bible clearly teaches that it's prideful to interrogate God about how He has made us. Such an attitude is dishonoring to God because it is an affront to His omniscience. Also, instead of bolstering our conviction that God knows what is best for each of our lives, it fosters regret and dissatisfaction over God's handiwork in our lives. Over time, we come to doubt God's ability to truly care for us and to bring good out of what may seem like needless pain or suffering. But even when we don't understand certain aspects of how God has made us, He desires us to implicitly trust that He has a master plan in place.

It's impossible to look at one or even a few pieces of a jigsaw puzzle and know what the puzzle is all about. Life is a lot like that. While we may be looking at one piece of our life and wondering how it could possibly fit into a beautiful plan, God can see and has seen the entire finished puzzle of our life; He knows not only where each piece goes but also the purpose that it serves because, again, He is all-wise and all-knowing.

From a very early age, my beloved mother often instructed my siblings and me "to never wish or desire to be the next man." This was her way of shielding us from that natural tendency to compare ourselves to others and to feel as though we don't measure up. She often quoted this maxim by Shakespeare: "All that glitters isn't gold." I'm so thankful that my dear mother laid this godly foundation in my formative years, long before I had an inkling of what it meant to live my life for God's glory, when I was as yet unaware that to embrace how God had made me—all of me, from the top of my head to the soles of my clubbed feet—is a very powerful expression of magnifying His worth.

IT'S YOURS ALONE—THERE'S NO NEED TO AUDITION!

God has uniquely designed each of us for a preordained purpose. Seek to internalize that truth. The Bible teaches that from eternity past, before there was either time or a universe, the triune God—Father, Son, and Holy Spirit—has always existed. The antithesis of this truth is that there was a point when there was no you and no me . . . nor anyone else for that matter. The Lord of the universe then skillfully shaped each person who has ever lived and put each one of us on the metaphorical grand stage of life. Biblical characters such as Abraham, Moses, Ruth, Joseph, Esther, Daniel, Naomi, Jonah, Hannah, and David each had a specific role to play. And so do you.

In a theatrical play, characters have differing roles and the script dictates when those characters appear onstage. From eternity past, God has developed the master script, not just for you and me but for an entire universe of people who have ever lived. He alone is the divine Director of our lives, determining when we each would appear on life's stage. So let the following sink in: you have a significant role, and it is God's will and plan that *your* appearance on the grand stage of life is *now*!

Unlike a Broadway play, however, there was no need for an audition. We should be awed that, even before time began, God had already cast each of us for our unique roles. Yet we must never lose sight of the fact that God doesn't need us (see Acts 17:24–25); He simply desires to work through us to advance His kingdom on the earth. We can willingly embrace our role or dig in our heels in an attempt to resist God's plan for our lives. God will either reward our obedience or we will suffer loss (of rewards) for our disobedience. (Eternal rewards are discussed more fully in Chapter 20.) Nevertheless, God is sovereign. We emphatically cannot derail His plans, and nothing or no one—not even Satan—can thwart His plans and purposes (see Isaiah 14:24, 27; 37:26, 44:7, 46:9–11; Psalm 115:3). In His omnipotence and unsearchable wisdom, God will sovereignly accomplish on earth all that He has purposed and ordained regardless of our level of participation or willingness to cooperate with His plans.

Similar to an actress who enjoys performing her given part, we must joyfully embrace the unique role that God's given us if we desire to live backward and make our lives count. In a sense, God desires us to "perform" on life's stage in a way that causes His name to be lifted up and exalted. Without question, the omniscient and renowned Producer of the universe desires each of our lives to be a rousing success. In one way or another, each one of us is truly one of God's star performers! How often we overlook this truth!

Let me ask you a question: Have you ever given any thought as to why you were born during *this particular* period of time? Why were you not born nine hundred years ago or three thousand years ago? What about sometime in the future? For that matter, why were you born *where* you were born? After all, God could have picked any of the ten thousand cities or towns in the world to be your birth place. The short answer is that you are treasured by your heavenly Father. And because He loves you with an everlasting love, He has planned out each and every detail of your life: the period of time that you'd exist, who your parents would be, right down to where you'd live. If you don't believe me, see Acts 17:26. Esther 4:14 says that Esther was born "for such a time as this"—and so are we.

Amid the clamor and distractions of life, though, we easily gloss over the exciting reality that God has uniquely created and designed each of us for a specific purpose. It's important that we really grasp these three realities: we are each designed perfectly by God to fulfill a unique plan, there's a vacuum in our hearts only God can satisfy, and we were born at a specific time and place by God's choosing. Together, these truths encapsulate what it means to contextualize one's life. The sad fact is that most people never make a difference because they simply fail to contextualize their lives, and in so doing, they fail to truly live.

FATHER OF OUR FAITH—NOT EXACTLY "HONEST ABE"

Part of this failure to contextualize our lives is rooted in our innate propensity to minimize or underestimate what God can accomplish through us and to focus on our flaws rather than celebrate the standout gifts that He has deposited in us. We undervalue what God has given us and overvalue what we think we don't have or lack. Conversely, we tend to magnify well-known biblical characters, viewing them as superheroes who easily achieved great things. We're tempted to believe that they somehow didn't have our weaknesses or experience the same struggles that we go through. We forget that they were nothing special—just ordinary people like you and me through whom God accomplished extraordinary things. As a matter of fact, many of them were quite messed up. Take for instance, Abraham, the father of our faith. He wasn't exactly Honest Abe. Not once but twice, Abraham contrived the same plan in a desperate attempt to save his life: he lied, saying Sarai was his sister not his wife so that a king could have sexual relations with her (see Genesis 12:11–19, 20:2).

But the plot thickens. Earlier God Himself had promised Abraham that Sarai would bear him a son, in spite of the fact that they were both well advanced in years. However, many years went by and Sarai still didn't bear any children. So she enjoins her husband to sleep with her maidservant, Hagar, in order to start a family. Surprisingly, or perhaps not so surprisingly, Abraham goes along with her request. Later, Sarai brazenly blames her husband for the tumultuous relationship that ensued between Hagar and herself (see Genesis 16:1–6). From what I've heard, the details and surprising twists and turns of this biblical account would seem to make fitting material for an episode of *Desperate Housewives of Egypt.*

AND A MURDERER SHALL LEAD US . . .

Or consider Moses. Let's not sugarcoat it . . . Moses committed a premeditated murder (see Exodus 2:11–12). Nevertheless, God called Moses from tending sheep and used him and his brother to deliver His chosen people out of Egyptian captivity. God accomplished this remarkable and amazing feat despite Moses's reluctance and self-perceived inadequacy (see Exodus 3:9–4:17). In fact, the entire book of Exodus is replete with miracle after miracle that God empowered Moses to perform while leading His people toward the Promised Land.

In addition, Moses questioned God, just as we have a tendency to do. When God told him to go and tell the Pharaoh of Egypt to let His people go, Moses doubted his ability and attempted to avoid God's call on his life (not once but on three different occasions). He claimed— better yet, he *told* God—that he was incapable of the task because he was "slow of speech and of tongue" (Exodus 4:10). The Lord's reply is stunningly humbling: "Who has made man's mouth? Who makes him mute, or deaf, or seeing, or blind? Is it not I, the Lord?" (Exodus 4:11). God has skillfully shaped each of us, and this account of Moses is but one of several that exemplify how God is more than able to accomplish whatever He desires through any of us.

ANOTHER MURDERER—NOT AGAIN

David, who is estimated to have authored more than seventy-eight Psalms, was also an Israelite king and ancestor of Jesus. However, David had some serious flaws as well. Let's take a peek into a telling period of his life. As David walked on his roof one evening, he caught sight of a beautiful woman named Bathsheba who was taking a bath. He sent his men to bring her to him even though he was duly informed that she was married to Uriah, a soldier in David's army. He proceeded to sleep with her, and she conceived a child. The drama intensifies. After David discovers that Bathsheba is carrying his child, he sends word to Joab, his commanding officer, to have Uriah sent home from battle. His scheme is simple but clever—to bring Uriah from the front lines so that he can sleep with Bathsheba and make it appear as though the child that she's carrying is his.

However, Uriah refused to sleep with his wife while his comrades were still facing danger. The following night, David "wines and dines" Uriah and gets him drunk as a last resort to get him to sleep with his wife. Again, Uriah refuses to lay with his wife. David resorts to a more desperate plan, sending Uriah back to the battle with a note to Joab instructing him to position Uriah at the front lines where the fighting is the fiercest and then withdraw from him so that he may be struck down. Sure enough, Uriah is killed. As soon as Bathsheba's time of mourning for her husband is over, David promptly brings her into his palace and marries her. She then bears him a son who subsequently dies after God strikes him with an illness (see 2 Samuel 11–12:18). Despite all this scheming and conniving, David is nevertheless referred to as "a man after God's own heart" (Acts 13:22).

YOU ARE OF IMMEASURABLE VALUE

For the sake of emphasis, let me ask you a couple of questions. Have you ever killed someone? If married, have you felt it was OK to conveniently give your spouse to another person for a few days so long as it served your own self-interests? Likely not. I've briefly summarized the above three accounts to underscore an often overlooked fact. Although we tend to place biblical characters on a pedestal, the superstars of the Bible were people with sins, flaws, insecurities, and weaknesses just like us, through whom God accomplished His plans and purposes (and there are many, many more, including Mary [the mother of Jesus], Sarai, Jephthah, Rahab, Jacob, and Gideon, to name just a few). Clearly, God empowered regular or ordinary people to do great things for Him! Our God still specializes in taking inadequate people and using them to demonstrate His power and His glory. Be filled with the hope that just as God used biblical characters in spite of their flaws, shortcomings, and failures, He wants to use you too! Our attitude should be: *if Abraham, Moses, David (and others) could fulfill their role in history with God's help, then so can I!* God is your Redeemer. There's nothing you have ever done or can ever do that can take Him or His promises away from you. God has promised to never leave us, fail us, or abandon us (see Deuteronomy 31:8). So don't give up on yourself and don't give up on God. Take to heart His wonderful assurance that He longs to be gracious and merciful to you (see Isaiah 30:18). Always remember that *you matter* and have immeasurable value to Him. You always have and you always will!

DISCOVERING OUR ROLE

Very briefly, we discover our roles when God-given passions and desires collide with a genuine need, or when they simply rouse us into action. These God moments and divine opportunities drive our sense of purpose. They open our eyes to how God wants to use us to make a difference and make an impact on the world for His glory. One of my favorite sayings is that your calling is where your passion meets your strength. Practically, the pursuit of our God-given passions should get us excited about getting out of bed in the morning and keep us from wanting to fall asleep at night. I have a friend, for instance, who could hardly sleep the night before he returned to work after a medical leave of absence because he missed doing what he loves. He is living his God-given purpose! My brother, an entrepreneur, has at times traversed three different continents within a matter of a few days. My family often kids that he spends more time in the air than he does on the ground. His demanding travel schedule would do most people in, but he doesn't mind it in the least because God has created him for this; he simply loves what he does.

EMBRACING OUR ROLE

The greatest love story ever told, the Bible unveils God's redemptive plan to restore all creation and all peoples back to complete enjoyment of Himself (see 1 Corinthians 15:28). It is a record of not only past events but also future prophecies, many of which have already been fulfilled. Yet in an entirely different sense, God's story—or *His*tory—is still being written today. Each and every one of us is part of this eternal, grand story. This means that the Creator of the entire universe and Author of life is still writing *your* life story. And He isn't through. No matter what it may look like now, God has a special plan for your life.

The biblical character Joseph must have at times felt as though God had placed him on a shelf and forgotten all about him. Despite doing all the right things (after being taken to Egypt and sold as a slave), Joseph was falsely accused of a crime and subsequently imprisoned for two years. Yet he eventually rose to prominence as second only to the Pharaoh of Egypt. Here's how my husband explains God's orchestration of the events in Joseph's life to ultimately bring good out of evil (see Genesis 39–45): "The end of his story is not the middle; never get lost in what the story is now, because it is not the end of the story." And it's the same for our lives. Like Joseph, maybe you can identify with the plight of disastrous circumstances, feeling useless or as though life is passing you by. However, God has promised to complete the good work that He has begun in each of us (see Philippians 1:6). When you grasp that He is always masterfully shaping you and sovereignly directing the countless scenes of your life, rather than worry you'll be able to experience the peace that surpasses all understanding, even in the midst of life's difficulties and storms (see Isaiah 26:3; Philippians 4:6–7).

You'll also come to deeply appreciate that the roles and scenes God has chosen for someone else is distinct from what He desires to do with your life for His glory. The simple truth is that we can greatly honor God simply by no longer comparing ourselves to others—by truly celebrating and employing the unique gifts He has given us for the display of His fame. As Oscar Wilde, the Irish poet and playwright once said, "Be yourself; everyone else is already taken."

We should embrace our roles knowing that, besides having written our individual scripts, God has graciously given us all the props and talents we need to succeed in whatever He has called us to do, be it on a large or small scale. God calls us to fervently pray for Him to do whatever He desires to do both in us and through us; to continually trust that what He has in store for us is best; to diligently seek His direction by following His divine GPS; and to patiently wait on His timetable, knowing that no matter the season—even if it takes a decade or a lifetime to fulfill—He will bring our life's purpose to fruition.

Be inspired! Get excited about living out your own unique story, walking in the freedom to boldly step out in faith for God! John Piper wisely states, "But whatever you do, find the God-centered, Christ-exalting, Bible-saturated passion of your life, and find your way to say it and live for it and die for it. And you will make a difference that lasts. You will not waste your life."[15] Living out such a life of passion for God should greatly inspire and motivate us.

So I implore you, adamantly refuse to simply go through the motions of life. Instead, pursue your God-given purpose. As sure as the sun rises in the east and sets in the west, God has given you a passion. Discover it. Contextualize it. Walk in it. Don't just exist, live! But *live backward.* Begin with the end firmly in mind—your "performance" on the grand stage of life is intended for nothing less than to delight the

---

15. John Piper, *Don't Waste Your Life* (Wheaton: Crossway, 2003), 47.

heart of God by bringing Him glory. I want to tell you that this impassioned pursuit of God is worth more than you can possibly fathom. Why? The answer bears repeating. Your "real" life begins when this one ends, and God has promised to eternally and handsomely reward those who live for His renown.

CHAPTER 4

······················

SERIOUS JOY

There is a kind of happiness and wonder that
makes you serious.
—C. S. Lewis

Many of us use technological gadgets without fully understanding how
they do what they do. For example, I typed the manuscript of this book
on a computer. In the process, I cut and pasted large portions of text
from one file to another; saved multiple versions of the Word file to
the hard drive, as well as uploaded them to the cloud; attached files
to e-mails which I then forwarded to others; and other similar tasks.
However, I cannot tell you how a computer's hardware or software
makes any of these seemingly complicated tasks possible. My lack of
computer knowledge doesn't damage the computer, for the most part;
neither does it limit my ability to use it efficiently or to reasonably
appreciate the wonderful things it can do for me.

I think we tend to view our relationship with God in a similar
way—we believe we can get along just fine in our spiritual life without
really knowing the attributes or inner workings of God. In actuality,
we can't.

The flip side of this analogy is also true. Similar to the more we know about computers, the more fully we can appreciate and maximize their benefits, so too the better we understand God, the more fully we can appropriate all that He desires us to experience. So the goal of this chapter is to explore some of God's awesome attributes because our grasp of them influences everything—from how we see and relate to God, to how we view His desires for our lives, to how we routinely go about our days.

For instance, comprehending the attribute of God's sheer awesomeness has helped to both shape in me and strengthen the God-centered view of life so vital to living for the praise of His glory. Practically speaking, we cannot truly find God worthy of our admiration and honor if we don't really know the essence of who He is, any more than we can appreciate the artistic ability of a painter without seeing any of her beautiful paintings. But knowing God is not just understanding who He is or comprehending His infinite greatness; it's also having a rock-solid confidence that He is closer to us and knows us better than even our spouse or best friend. To live with this awareness is to tap into a rich source of comfort, security, boldness, and freedom as we navigate the journey of life.

KNOWN SINCE ETERNITY PAST

My heart deeply resonates with the quote at the beginning of this chapter. I've discovered there is indeed a type of joy that makes one serious. In His goodness, God has graciously given me something simple yet priceless: a desire to seek Him. For many years now, I've earnestly sought to know the God of the universe who not only created me but also knew me before I was even conceived. Truly, God's knowledge of us is unfathomable! I am awed that even before the foundations of the earth were established, God not only saw me but knew me by name. I marvel that He arranged the day and time of my birth and has always known exactly where I'd take my very first breath.

Of course, the same applies to you. As we've seen, God's astonishing workmanship in our lives showcases our immeasurable worth to Him. Besides carefully and wondrously knitting together each and every aspect of our physical features, personality, and temperament, as well as endowing each of us with unique gifts and abilities of His precise choosing (see Ephesians 4:7), God has planted dreams and desires in us so that we may lead fulfilling lives that exalt Him. God is also inexpressibly involved in our lives. He has preordained the number of our days on the earth (see Psalm 39:4). How incredulous that God knows the number of hairs on our head and is aware of our thoughts before we even speak (see Luke 12:7; Psalm 139:2). He is intimately acquainted with everything about us, right down to the minutest detail—our deepest thoughts, fears, quirks, likes, dislikes, pet peeves, and restless longings. God knows the deepest wound and heartache we will ever experience in this life. Likewise, He also knows each and every life event that will make our hearts swell with joy.

GOD DOES NOT WEAR A WATCH

I could go on and on about God's wisdom and how intimately He knows each of us (see Isaiah 40 for a beautiful description of God's wisdom and sovereignty). From eternity past, God *knows*, *knew*, always *has known*, and always *will know* everything there is to know about you and me. He holds our past, present, and future in His capable and omnipotent hands.

However, with God, there is no continuum labeling past, present, or future. God does not need a timepiece, for He dwells outside the finite dimensions or limitations of time and space. Although it's difficult for us to grasp, God's existence is somehow always present. In other words, He dwells in an eternal present. God sees everything (or everything exists) as the present. This is why Jesus Christ could declare, "Before Abraham was, I am" (John 8:58). God knows what He has always known and forever will know about the entire universe, including this grand stage on which we live. This awesome attribute of God's timelessness substantiates why biblical prophecies declared thousands of years ago have been, and continue to be, fulfilled.

To make this practical, God sees the years 2020 BC, 600 BC, AD 850, AD 1715, AD 1982, AD 2027 (assuming the Lord tarries His return) and every year—past, present, and future—all at the same time! Mind-boggling, isn't it? If God sees our present, past, and future through the lens of His Eternal Present, think of its profound implications relating to His loving and attentive care for us. The reason God can govern each and everything that enters our lives *and* cause them all to work together for our good (see Romans 8:28) is precisely *because* He knows or sees the past, present, and future all at the same time. When we can't see them, God already sees the wonderful things He has in store for us. For example, when I felt overwhelmed and crushed during my pregnancy losses, God already saw me holding, feeding, and nurturing the three children He would subsequently bring into my life; it was just a matter of time before I'd experience these sweet blessings. We can trust that God hears the prayers of His children (see Proverbs 15:29; Psalm 34:15, 17; 1 Peter 3:12) and will give us His good gifts at His appointed time, not a millisecond too soon or too late.

Similarly, when a horrific or tragic event befalls one generation, God already knows how He will use it as a catalyst or stepping-stone for later generations to not just thrive but flourish. An example of this is the Great Migration, which lasted from World War I to the 1970s and changed the face of America. Over this period, some six million black Americans left behind the cruel and harsh inequities of the South, fanning out to points north and west in search of a better way of life. As a result of this uprooting and transplanting, children, grand-children, and great-grandchildren of these migrants were afforded the opportunity to pursue their dreams and achieve success beyond what their forebears could have ever imagined possible. Isabel Wilkerson, author of *The Warmth of Other Suns*, which brilliantly chronicles this watershed moment in US history, speaks about the famous children of these migrants:

> Many famous Americans were products of the Great Migration, and there's no way to know what their lives might have been like or if their achievements would have been possible had it not been for the courage of the parents or grandparents who left the South. Each of them grew up to become among the best in their fields, changed them, really. They were among the first generation of blacks in this country to grow up free and unfettered because of the actions of parents or grandparents who knew it was not too late for their children.[16]

While absolutely not minimizing the persistent, far-reaching ramifications of its cruel and abhorrent social injustices, God brought good even out of a caste system as atrocious and denigrating as slavery. Life indeed is not fair. But God—the God of justice and vindication—has given us His unalterable word that someday He will right every wrong that His children have ever experienced on this fallen earth (see Psalm 37:12–13; Ecclesiastes 3:17): physical and emotional pain, handicaps, and every wicked thing—wars, inequities, persecution, oppression, calamity—will be no more, for He Himself will wipe away every tear from our eyes.

What about eternity? Have you ever thought about the fact that even now God sees you bedazzled by Heaven's splendor, capable of doing things so wondrous that you can't even dare to conceive? God's omniscience, along with His omnipresence, goodness, and providence, should fill us with heartfelt thanksgiving and grateful praise.

---

16. Isabel Wilkerson, "Author Interview," accessed February 18, 2015, http:// isabelwilkerson.com/about/author-interview/.

WE CAN TRUST GOD WITH OUR LIVES

Because of these unshakable aspects of God's nature, there's never a time that He isn't mindful of us. Despite evidence seemingly to the contrary, where it may seem as if God is not omnipotent, God controls the broad strokes of human history as well as our individual lives. He never misses a single thing! Scripture assures us that nothing escapes God's notice: "What is the price of two sparrows—one copper coin? But not a single sparrow can fall to the ground without your Father knowing it. And the very hairs on your head are all numbered. So don't be afraid; you are more valuable to God than a whole flock of sparrows" (Matthew 10:29–31, New Living Translation). Think about it: the same omnipotent God who simply spoke all of creation into existence and who upholds the entire universe by the word of His power also (see Hebrews 1:3) holds each of our lives. Therefore, we can entrust ourselves to His faithful care. Proverbs 3:5–6 tells us, "Trust in the Lord with all your heart, and do not lean on your own understanding. In all your ways acknowledge him, and he will make straight your paths." Yet just like we're unable to trust a stranger or someone we barely know, it's very difficult to place our trust in God if we don't understand His character. This brings us back to the importance of knowing what God has revealed of Himself in His Word.

Furthermore, this trust doesn't develop overnight; it's certainly a process. Generally, we start off trusting God with relatively small concerns, for example, that He would allow a specific check to arrive before the anticipated time. When the check indeed gets to you a week earlier than expected, your trust in God goes up a notch. When subsequently faced with a bigger challenge, like being told you're not eligible for the raise that you were desperately counting on, you recall how God previously moved on your behalf. You pray and trust Him to make a way out of what seems to be no way. When you receive a larger sum of money—for instance, an insurance reimbursement—completely out of the blue, your trust doesn't just go up another notch, it experiences a growth spurt. Each time we see God move on our behalf, in both the big and little things, it builds up our trust in Him. Again and again, we can look back and see His faithfulness.

Besides trusting our heavenly Father with situations such as the above, we can trust Him with all the intricate details of our lives simply because He holds each and every moment of our lives in His all-wise and all-powerful hands. Because God is never caught off guard or surprised by anything that we experience, whether small or significant, we can also have the utmost confidence in knowing that nothing ever enters our lives that hasn't first been filtered through His omniscience and great love for us. Nothing just happens without a reason, so we don't have to worry about anything that the future holds; we don't have to be enslaved to fear of the unknown. Several Scriptures attest to this truth that God is in control of *all* things. Not only does He do all that He pleases, God knows the end from the beginning, and as I've mentioned, nothing or no one can thwart His plans and purposes. By the same token, there's also no such thing as coincidence—God's hands are in everything. Scripture is clear: "We may throw the dice, but the LORD determines how they fall" (Proverbs 16:33, New Living Translation). If nothing in this universe happens by mere coincidence, then the same is true of luck. Hence, a simple but very powerful way to magnify God's glory is to *never* ascribe as luck or coincidence anything that He graciously bestows on us. To do so is a grievous affront not only to God's goodness toward us but also to His honor. In the same vein, nothing comes into our lives as a result of bad luck.

God wants us to rest in the knowledge that He mysteriously uses all our varied circumstances to fulfill His plans and purpose for our lives, even the difficult ones that often seem to make absolutely no sense. I want you to really get this incredible truth about God's sovereignty because it largely determines the degree to which you'll experience His joy, peace, and contentment as you engage this life: God has *always* known the countless, cascading life experiences that you'll have; He has orchestrated them to shape you into the individual He desires you to be. And He desires you to take Him at His word. Ultimately, not a single detail about your life is without purpose! When we really get this truth, we are empowered to completely trust God with everything concerning our lives.

Father—our heavenly Father, that is—truly knows best! For example, He knows how a tragic car accident a person sustained ten years ago would work in concert with the loss of a job three years later to help bring that person to the end of himself, causing him or her to cry out to God. He is a God of restoration and has always known how He would redeem or recycle these two circumstances into something good. Scripture affirms this reality: "To all who mourn in Israel, he will give a crown of beauty for ashes, a joyous blessing instead of mourning, festive praise instead of despair" (Isaiah 61:3, New Living Translation). I've learned that often our setbacks are setups in disguise, which God uses to do a deeper work in our lives and prepare us for something greater. So instead of feeling defeated, wallowing in self-pity, or losing hope, we can be assured that even though we can't see what God is up to, He is nevertheless attentively at work in our lives and has good things in store. God is like a matchless weaver who sees the entire tapestry of each of our lives—He knows the precise timing and exactly how to weave every single thread in order to bring about the beautiful masterpieces He has envisioned from eternity past. How different would our outlook be if we truly believed and lived out this truth!

I've learned (and continue to learn) that when I remember to pause and see God's divine orchestration in all things . . . life amazingly takes on a profound simplicity. As we progressively learn to accept each and every situation in our lives as ultimately coming from God for *His glory and our greatest good*, regardless of how significant or insignificant, how big or small, we begin to view all of life through God-centered lens. The result is that we truly become different people who see trials, failures, challenging circumstances, setbacks, defeats, irritations, and frustrations in an entirely new light and from a radically different perspective—His.

The practical benefits of this God-centered perspective are wonderful. For example, I tend to be impatient while driving. More and more, I am less bothered about missing a green light or that someone in front of me on a one-lane road is driving too slowly when I remember that God just might have a reason. Instead of being flustered, I can be at peace and rejoice that He may have allowed these irritations to help me avoid a potential accident, perhaps only a few seconds later. This awareness fortifies my trust that God is in control and is vigilantly watching over me. Besides enlarging our ability to more fully trust God—both in the mundaneness of life and in carrying out His unique purpose for our lives—a God-centered perspective progressively empowers us to tap into the boundless grace that Christ died for us to obtain. Grace sustains us, strengthens us, emboldens us, builds our faith and hope, makes us overcomers, fills us with joy, and anchors us in peace—there's no end to what the abounding grace of God can accomplish in our lives.

I don't think there's a person alive who would say, "I can't use more peace in my life." We can experience this peace because God promises peace to His people (see Psalm 85:8). In fact, Jesus *is* the Prince of Peace (see Isaiah 9:6), and since He lives within us, we just need to believe it by faith and learn to access it. Although it eludes many of us, knowing how to walk in God's peace is not a secret. Actually, it's quite simple: the more deeply we understand and embrace God's sovereign orchestration of our lives, the more deeply we'll also experience His abiding peace. Experiencing and showing forth God's peace would do wonders for our testimony in a world that is in constant turmoil and confusion.

GOD IS TOO MARVELOUS FOR COMPREHENSION

The knowledge that the most high God is always sovereignly orchestrating or weaving all the events in our lives, not only for His glory but also for our ultimate good (to the end of conforming us to Christ) should also fill us with great hope. We should be greatly encouraged that today as well as each and every day in the future, our omnipotent God has promised to attentively watch over us because He deeply cares about us and longs to show us compassion.

The God we serve, the King of Kings and Lord of Lords who desires us to live for Him, is too awesome for words! He's too marvelous for comprehension! When indeed we are overtaken by His loving kindness toward us, our hearts will resonate with David's exclamation, "Such knowledge is too wonderful for me; it is high; I cannot attain it . . . How precious to me are your thoughts, O God! How vast is the sum of them! If I would count them, they are more than the sand . . ." (Psalm 139:6, 17–18). Like David was, I am overwhelmed that though the infinite, all-powerful, and all-knowing God "sits above the circle of the earth" (Isaiah 40:22) and sovereignly governs all life, He is not distant from me. Rather, He is closer to me than the very air I breathe because incredibly, He has chosen to make my heart His dwelling place.

Even more awe-inspiring, not only is God governing all the immeasurable events in our lives, He is simultaneously orchestrating the immeasurable events—which are never static but always dynamic—in the lives of the billions and billions of people who now live, have lived, and will ever live. This is even more incomprehensible when we consider the limitless ways that all the aggregate details and events in the life of just one person can potentially intersect with an infinite number of other persons, places, events, and circumstances. It's simply incredulous! "Oh, the depth of the riches and wisdom and knowledge of God! How unsearchable are his judgments and how inscrutable his ways" (Romans 11:33). This truth humbles me and fills me with awe.

LONGING FOR A RELATIONSHIP WITH ME?

The glorious truth that the sovereign God of the universe not only loves me but has always loved me and longs to have an intimate relationship with me overwhelms me to the core. It makes me plain ecstatic that the all-sufficient God who is in need of nothing outside Himself, the God who is indeed Everything—knows everything, made everything, does everything He pleases, and *has* everything—nevertheless *still desires me.* I believe nothing else should more captivate a child of God. Therefore, the joy that this awareness should engender ought to be the kind that makes one, well, serious!

Such it has done for me. There is now nothing of greater importance in my life than seeking, by the power of the Holy Spirit, to know this awesome God who passionately loves me. I desire to wholeheartedly love Him in return. In trying to describe the zeal that God has birthed in me, I sincerely do not want to come off as overly pious or spiritual. I assure you, even though I know that the blood of Christ has once and for all made me clean and righteous in God's sight, no one needs to tell me that sinful desires and old thought patterns still lurk in my heart. I am keenly aware that I continually fall short of demonstrating God's character. Nevertheless, I sincerely desire that each beat of my heart would increasingly long to be in concert with His.

BY-PRODUCTS OF SEEKING GOD

I trust this acknowledgment of my sinful tendencies will be the lens through which you view the following examples of how God has changed my desires, realigned my priorities, reshaped my thinking, and radically transformed my life as I've grown in my understanding of Him: I find myself preoccupied with knowing God better, and the more I know Him, the more I long to love Him even more. I've become very mindful that it's quite difficult to know Jesus and the fellowship of His suffering so long as I seek to live within the confines of my safe and comfortable Christian bubble. In fact, I'm at this moment very uncomfortable about feeling so comfortable, resulting in a gnawing righteous discontent not being spent enough for the kingdom of God. I'm desperate for my life to conform more and more to the example of Christ.

On the practical side, my life is pretty much free of anxiety and worry as I rest in the certainty that God is in control of every event and situation that I face. Admittedly, I often forget to pray for my temporal needs because I'm praying instead for more of God's presence and power in my life. Overcome by God's goodness, I have found that more and more my thoughts instinctively turn toward Him, and throughout the day I lift my heart to Him in spontaneous praise. Standing in awe of God and living for His glory doesn't benefit only me, it is of great benefit to my relationships with others as well. For example, as my husband and I choose to make God foremost in our lives—dying daily to fleshly desires, pursuing holiness, and putting each other's needs ahead of our own—we've enjoyed a loving, intimate, and grace-filled marriage that truly gets better and better with each passing year, and we treasure the tender and beautiful relationships with each of the three children God has entrusted to us. Besides making me a better wife and parent, earnestly seeking to magnify Christ strengthens all my relationships and positively affects how I relate to every single person with whom I interact.

I almost hesitate to add that eating more than I truly need, eating when I'm not hungry, or just having too large of a portion to begin with no longer masters me. Besides breathing, nothing in our lives is more basic than eating and drinking. Yet even in these things we are called to glorify God as 1 Corinthians 10:31 teaches: "So whether you eat or drink, or whatever you do, do *all* to the glory of God" (emphasis mine). I'm very grateful that God continues to help me not be a slave to my stomach, giving it whatever it wants, whenever it wants it. The wonderful by-product of my desire to honor God in all aspects of my life, even in my eating, is that I've maintained my desired weight for more than a decade now. It is truly remarkable how God has faithfully and lovingly changed me.

DROWNING IN GRACE

Through continually pressing in to seek, know, and love God more, He has brought me to a sweet place of intimacy with Him. For a very long time, this place seemed so far off, even unattainable. What exactly characterizes "this place"? Well, let me first say what it is not. It's not a place where there is superficial love for God because of the exceedingly plentiful gifts He has generously bestowed. If that were the case, it would mean that I desire God's gifts more than I desire Him. May that never be so! How empty my life would be if I were seeking the output of God's grace versus intimacy with my Maker, Himself!

What if God in His providence were to take His gifts—family, health, finances, and so on—away from us? Would we still love Him? Better still, if God desired us to *willingly* relinquish that which we love and cherish—for instance, a job, vehicle, home, or career—would we be offended and turn our backs on Him? At some point in our faith journey, we must each ask ourselves these questions. The latter, in particular, is worthy of honest and serious reflection because the thing that we are least willing to part with has the greatest potential to ensnare us—to vie for our loyalty to Jesus or even become a substitute for Him. That's why Jesus adamantly calls us to surrender all that we are and all that we have in order to follow Him. He emphatically taught, "Whoever loves father or mother more than me is not worthy of me, and whoever loves son or daughter more than me is not worthy of me. And whoever does not take his cross and follow me is not worthy of me. Whoever finds his life will lose it, and whoever loses his life for my sake will find it" (Matthew 10:37–39). There's simply no way that we can bring glory to God while seeking to live for ourselves and forward our own agendas.

Hence, "this place" is a sweet spot where having willingly surrendered what I had envisioned for my life to God—all my hopes, dreams, and desires—I found the freedom to truly live. It's a place born of a burning desire to walk upright before God and to be more holy, both in the meditations of my heart and in my overall attitude and conduct (see Psalm 139:23). It represents a point in my spiritual journey where my will to selfishly live for myself became eclipsed by my desire to keep a continual smile on my Father's face. This heart posture continues to sink me deeper into the oceans of God's grace, compelling me to delight in Him more and more. As I gulp in His love and grace, my ever-grateful heart revels and dances in the sheer delight my Father takes in me as His precious daughter.

LIVING IN THE DIVINE SPOTLIGHT

The offshoot of this glorious place is that I'm more cognizant that my life is ever being lived out before an "audience of one." Because of this heightened awareness of living in God's presence, I realize that at any given moment my choices, motives, decisions, and actions are either pleasing Him or grieving His indwelling Spirit. Far from being dreadful, however, living in the divine spotlight makes me keenly aware that everything I do—even in the nitty-gritty, mundane moments of life— can and indeed should become worship unto the Lord. This awareness fosters a greater desire to please God in every way. It also provides countless teachable moments for the Holy Spirit to guide me, prick my conscience, correct me, warn me when I'm about to fall into a snare, encourage me, and convey His pleasure for my obedience. In short, I experience a special joy in those precious moments when I know that my life is delighting the heart of my Creator and King.

The fact that the world would think it both ludicrous and ironic that someone could derive any joy or pleasure from the knowledge that God's "terrible" eye is ever on His creatures can potentially be a teaching point for us to dialogue about how and why God governs all of His creation. Those in spiritual darkness understandably cannot comprehend that God's providential care—His watchful eye ever resting on His children—is one of the sweetest truths in His Word. The fact that the sovereign God of the universe justly but uncapriciously controls each and every aspect of our lives can and should be of great reassurance in an evil and fallen world. This truth means that ultimately nothing or no one, not even the devil himself, has the power to sabotage or derail God's plans and purposes for those who are His. Besides promoting my devotion to my heavenly Father, His attentive care strengthens my sense of nearness to Him.

I'm persuaded that first standing in awe of God and then living in His presence can fill each of us with an incredible sense of joy and peace—the kind of joy that indeed makes one serious.

CHAPTER 5

....

THE FALSE STRUGGLE

Each of our lives is like an instrument that
only God can teach us how to play.
—Jason Alvarado

PLAYING HIDE-AND-SEEK WITH SIGNIFICANCE

Have you at times questioned where you are in life? Ever felt
apprehensive that if life were a juicy orange, you're not really squeezing
out all the juice? I have. Even though I was awed by the indescribable
immensity of God and His great love for me, I nevertheless came to a
place where I felt as though I was missing out on some of His plans for
my life. Most everyone played hide-and-seek as a youngster. During
this time of searching, I felt like I was playing hide-and-seek with
the idea of my temporal significance. Truth be told, I didn't know if
I should have been hiding from the idea of significance or seeking to
explore it. I've since learned that it's critical to understand how seeking
fulfillment meshes with the idea of living backward to bring God glory.

I've always intuitively known (as a gift of God's grace) that God
does what He does so that His plans for my life may be accomplished.

I also recognized that the godly desires that the Holy Spirit stirred up in me were so that Christ would be magnified in my life. However, several years ago, while journaling and reflecting on my life, I suddenly realized that along with these godly desires, something else had welled up in me: namely, a seemingly latent yet growing desire for meaning or significance.

This revelation had caught me by surprise. *Significance in what?* I wondered. You see, although I had certain aspirations, I had already experienced a sense of fulfillment by achieving two things I had greatly desired: becoming a wife and mother. Moreover, I understood that, ultimately, God wanted me to find my truest significance and identity in the revelation of who I was as His child. As far as I could tell, He had enabled me to grasp this truth quite well. Besides, just the thought of the word "significance" conjured up a certain sense of "worldly self-importance" that I desired to completely avoid. I vaguely connected this desire with pride, and, at this point in my spiritual growth, God had worked into me a reverential fear of this pervasive sin deeply entrenched in all our hearts. An ancient foe, pride predates the fall of man, as it was this deadly sin which caused Eve to succumb to the enemy's temptation and to eat of the fruit that God had forbidden her and her husband from eating in the Garden of Eden. And even before the garden, it was pride that precipitated Satan's expulsion from his favored place in Heaven (see Ezekiel 28:12–17; Luke 10:18). Since then, pride has been contending for supremacy over God.

Furthermore, I was keenly aware that the very nature of pride is to subtly cloak itself so that we're often unable to discern its giant footprints all over our lives. The irony of pride, then, is that it is a sin that we can always seem to find in others but seldom see in ourselves. If sinful tendencies were likened to a storm, then pride is the eye.

Because pride seems to be at the root of all sin, I knew that by keeping it at bay, we could prevent a multitude of other sins from taking root in our hearts. I also knew firsthand that whether intentional or unintentional, overt or subtle, we are generally far more concerned about promoting our own honor than we are God's renown; we often set aside God's revealed will in order to advance our personal goals and interests and thereby receive the accolade and praise that we selfishly desire. In a sense, we desire to make ourselves bigger than God—we want to matter more than we want God to matter. This self-exaltation usurps God's rightful, blood-bought place on the throne of our hearts; and because God alone is deserving of all the glory, honor, and praise, pride is one of the most serious affronts against a holy and awesome God. Therefore, I took to heart this stern warning: "Everyone who is arrogant in heart is an abomination to the Lord" (Proverbs 16:5). For all these reasons, I wanted to avoid pride at all costs.

So as I pondered what this desire for significance could mean, I became perplexed. I even developed a spiritual angst of sorts. For some reason, I had come to earnestly believe that a desire for significance in some other area of my life—whatever it may look like—was at worst narcissistic and at best spiritually unhealthy. In fact, I thought this budding desire for significance was a strategic weapon of the enemy to appeal to my pride and subtly undermine my humility before God. So I quickly brushed aside the whole idea of significance.

A FALLACY REVEALED

Then God began to challenge my thinking. Prior to my discovery of this desire for significance, I had been very serious about conforming my life to Christ. However, I had not understood that God desires us to *actively* pursue great things for His kingdom. While the pursuit of Christlikeness is indeed our core purpose or destiny, God desires us to be an integral part of what He is doing on the earth to advance His glory. Ephesians 2:10 clearly teaches, "For we are his workmanship, created in Christ Jesus for good works, which God prepared beforehand, that we should walk in them." I must emphasize that this reference to "works" is not about vain, misdirected attempts to earn right standing with God. Scripture reveals that this is absolutely not possible (see Isaiah 64:6; Romans 10:3). "Works" here refers to those things God has appointed for us to do to advance His kingdom. Unbeknownst to me, I was so preoccupied with my pursuit of Christlikeness, I had become somewhat passive about pursuing those good works that God had ordained for me.

Thankfully, God began to open up my understanding. I discovered that our desire for significance culminates in who we are as God's image bearers, a people called to magnify His name and display His glory. Therefore, you and I can't help but yearn for significance. Whether we realize it or not, God has written eternity on each of our hearts (see Ecclesiastes 3:11). This Scripture suggests that, at least in one sense, God has shaped each of our hearts to desire enduring significance. This reality made much sense to me and transformed my perspective. I then started to embrace that my Father wanted me to diligently pursue conformity to Christ *and* actively seek to make His name great. Previously, I had not grasped that a willingness—no, better still, a passion—to seek out ways to make God's name great on earth was foundational to a life lived for His glory.

This is not to say that God isn't already famous, for all of creation testifies to His great power and awesome majesty. Rather, I'm speaking about having an expectant desire to be used of God to influence the world—in art, music, education, media, nonprofit, government, sports, business, civic groups, and religious organizations— however He desires. Up until this time, I simply hadn't been cultivating this desire. I soon realized that this area of passivity in my spiritual walk meant that I was not seeking to fully walk out God's plan for my life. I know that many other people are like I used to be, seeking Christlikeness in their desire to glorify God but not fully understanding that purposefully seeking out avenues to make His name great is integral to living for His glory.

My apprehension that God desires His children to actively seek to promote His fame soon raised some concerns. If followers of Christ do understand that we are called to passionately pursue God's honor, are we doing so? As His ambassadors, are we truly open to God's will for our lives, knowing that with Him absolutely nothing is impossible (see 2 Corinthians 5:20; Matthew 19:26; Mark 10:27; Luke 1:37)? Why do so many of us live seemingly indifferent to the truth that God desires to accomplish more through us than we could even dare imagine (see Ephesians 3:20)? We see this attitude manifest when we covet other people's strengths rather than embrace our own, minimize or shrug off a sincere compliment about a God-given talent or gift, or use our short-comings or our past to place limits on what God can do through us. To take this a step further, do we, as God's privileged children, believe that He can accomplish *anything* He desires through *anyone* He chooses to use? Do we engage life recognizing that God could empower any individual—you, me, your neighbor, a friend, the mailman, the children He's entrusted to you, absolutely anyone—to accomplish great and marvelous things for His kingdom?

Practically speaking, the world is full of evil and darkness. The fields are ripe for harvest. God is looking for present-day Obadiahs, the name that means "servant of the Lord." Are His children truly willing to live for Him and to serve Him? But lest we mistakenly think it necessary to traverse thousands of miles to serve as a missionary in a faraway country, we are missionaries or agents of change right where God has us. As the saying goes, "Bloom where you are planted." Whether it's something as far-reaching as what Martin Luther accomplished in the Reformation, going on a missions trip to another country to help the sick and poor, helping out at a local food pantry, or just giving a cup of water or a meal to someone in need, God wants to use His people to accomplish His work on earth.

AVOIDING PRIDE

The Holy Spirit helped me realize I had given only mental assent to the truth that God's children can accomplish anything for Him that He wants. Consequently, I wasn't embracing it in my life. In fact, you're reading this book because I wanted to—no, needed to—become unshackled from a lie I had believed for far too long.

For a lengthy period of time, I allowed my sincere desire for humility (and Christlikeness) to negate the possibility that God may desire to use me in a way that I perhaps could not even envision. The following statement might even sound foolish to you, but because I keenly recognized how pervasive and pernicious pride can be, I believed that if God did accomplish a particular good work through me, it would likely undermine the humility I so desperately sought. Aware that the Bible does teach us to be cautious about both the covert and overt manifestations of pride, I had mistakenly bought into the enemy's lie that my desire to fulfill God's unique plans for my life could not coexist with my desire to walk humbly before Him. Without knowing it, I had falsely internalized that growth in humility and the active pursuit of making God's name great (which should be woven into our desire for a life of significance) were somehow mutually exclusive—although, we still must be careful to avoid letting our pursuit of holiness morph into the pursuit of man's praise for ourselves rather than for God's glory. This perception of mutual exclusivity is, by the way, an example of the enemy's cunning attempts to abort God's plans for our lives.

I also knew how easy it is to become puffed up and to trust in one's own ability rather than depend on God. Yet, while distrust of my abilities was thankfully working to keep me humble, it was at the same time causing me to shrink back from a task that I sensed God wanted to do through me: namely, to write the book you are now reading.

Throughout this time the desire to write this book was always there, but I was reluctant about actually pursuing it. At times, I justified my complacency by recalling the importance of pursuing humility. Thankfully, however, I also wanted to know for certain that my desire for this writing project was truly from God—that it wasn't just a fleshly aspiration, as I want to obediently pursue the God things for my life, not the good or even the great things that are outside of His plans for me. I also recognized that, in addition to being the God thing, writing the book had to be aligned with God's timing. I've found that somewhere along this obedience and timing continuum, it's very easy to slip into passivity and rationalize why we aren't doing what we sense God is calling us to do.

LOOKING AT ONLY ONE SIDE OF THE COIN

At any rate, since I had foolishly reasoned that I couldn't pursue the desire or "good work" of writing this book and cultivate humility at the same time, I quite naturally concluded that I'd pursue only one of them. And in wanting to please God above all else, I erroneously figured that the godly choice would be to dismiss the desire to write a book and continue to pursue humility. Although I needed to be wary of the perniciousness of pride—which can beset us even when we're pursuing the God thing in our lives—my prudent, vigilant thinking represented only one side of the coin.

There is nothing prideful about pursuing our God-given dreams and aspirations. The truth is that humbly doing what God has called and equipped us to do (within the confines of His will and timing) not only glorifies God as we've seen but also brings Him joy and delight. In fact, just as it is prideful to question how God has made us, to intentionally ignore the calling God has placed on your life is a form of pride if your attitude amounts to telling God you know better than He what is best for your life. To purposefully not pursue your calling is to spurn the gifts God has entrusted to you, which dishonors Him. Attempting to evade being used of God (think Moses or Jonah!) is not humility at all; it is actually rebellion. (This statement, of course, excludes those times when we haven't yet discerned God's will for our lives.)

Now I know I can pursue humility and God's call on my life. I'm very grateful God enabled the desire He planted in my heart to write this book to eventually win out over my erroneous thinking, encouraging me, at the same time, to continue my pursuit of humility. Yet, as I write these words, my heart is grieved for having entertained small thoughts of our infinitely big and awesome God. While I was attempting to avoid pride, I overlooked the amazing truth that a God who is infinite also has infinite power at His disposal. Indeed, He has the wisdom, power, and might to supply anyone truly seeking Him with the requisite grace he or she needs to honor Him without compromising his/her humility.

I've heard similar stories of why others have shrunk back from pursuing God's call on their lives. I've shared this part of my story for the benefit of those who may have experienced deception in a similar vein. If you have, I want to encourage you to not become paralyzed or complacent about pursuing the good works God desires to accomplish through you for any reason, be it your pursuit of humility (as with me), a healthy fear of pride, feelings of inadequacy, the fear of letting God down in a specific task, fear in general, and so on.

EXTENSIVE SURGERY

In retrospect I now recognize that the above experience was part of the refining process I needed to go through to be better equipped to write this book. There was a time many years ago when I sensed it was God's plan for me to write a book on some aspect of Christian living. In my masked pride and self-confidence, I had believed myself fully capable of the task; I had felt completely confident in *my* ability to write a book. During this time, God began to perform surgery on my prideful heart. Over the subsequent years, He made me more pliable in His hands, transforming me from the inside out. A key result of this makeover was that the sins I came to see most starkly were those within my own heart. Should the Lord tarry or I'm not called home soon, the extensive surgery still required on my heart seems light-years from being over.

However, as a result of this spiritual surgery, God amazingly wrought in me a keen understanding of my desperate need for His transforming grace. As God worked this understanding into me, He also mercifully emptied me of much of the confidence I had in my own abilities, enabling me to see my great need to depend on Him all the more. Over time, the fanciful notion that I could write a book began to gradually lose its substance.

In fact, as I look back, I realize that I had imperceptibly started to believe that writing this book was perhaps not part of God's plan for my life after all. It was, but God needed to first humble me. And He sovereignly used even the whispered lie of the enemy—intended to short-circuit His plan for my life—to move me forward. While I mistakenly internalized that I couldn't pursue God's plans for my life and continue to remain humble, God was using that very period of time to humble me all the more.

Then it happened.

REVERSAL OF CONFIDENCE

Call it an epiphany . . . an indelible God moment! In the middle of a very ordinary day—while standing at the kitchen sink washing dishes and communing with God—something wonderful happened. It was a sacred moment of grace! The notion that I could write a book suddenly fizzled out like a fallen star. I was jolted into the realization that I was *utterly* incapable of writing a book. God had humbled me to the point where I felt completely daunted by just the mere thought of it. What a reversal!

A wistful sense of relief then washed over me as I thought, *Well, since I'm incapable of writing a book, I'm off the hook now for writing one!* Only, this was a fleeting thought. For in the next moment, it suddenly dawned on me that in God's economy of preparation or usefulness, this divestiture of self-confidence in my ability to write a book—which He had mysteriously bestowed upon me—now ironically made me an ideal candidate to author a book on Christian discipleship.

I was momentarily stunned as the thoughts of what this might actually mean flashed through my mind. Having authored a small book of poetry years earlier, I knew implicitly the huge demands on time, energy, and effort that writing a nonfiction book of this nature would entail. So the momentary "spiritual brain freeze" quickly gave way to a sense of panic that perhaps God really did want me to write a book after all.

A BIG FIRE LIT UNDER A SMALL POT

Have you ever had one of those moments when it seems God inaudibly whispers something to your heart, yet it's so clear that you know without a doubt He's "speaking" to you? That's exactly what I experienced in that moment at the kitchen sink; I just knew in my spirit that I had been called by God to write this book. And the time was now! God gave me an unbelievable passion and indescribable reserves of energy while writing. Instead of working up the energy to write, I experienced the exact opposite—time and time again I reluctantly had to pull myself away from the computer in order to fulfill my other responsibilities. I often skipped meals as I didn't feel hungry. I also didn't want to go to bed at night, often writing into the wee hours of the morning and at times going to bed after the sun had risen; each day I couldn't wait to continue working. And this went on for well over three and a half years! There's absolutely no way that I humanly could have mustered up this type of energy and drive over such a protracted period of time.

Only a supernatural God can energize and empower someone in such an incredible way. For me this most intense drive was confirmation that I was in the center of His will.

God has ignited a big fire under my very small pot. Roaring and ablaze, it has caused my small pot to boil over with zeal for God's glory and renown. Were I not to write this book, this burning zeal—like "fire shut up in my bones"—threatened to consume me. My hope is that God will use this book to ignite another big fire under a different small pot. In time, I hope this other pot will also begin to boil over with zeal for God's glory. If such a fire is lit under just one brother or sister in Christ, whose zeal in turn influences another small pot to boil over with zeal for God, then this book would have accomplished its objective. Why? Simply because our Lord and King has called us to carry out the Great Commission. Intrinsic to this command is to go and make other disciples, baptizing them in the name of the Father and of the Son and of the Holy Spirit (see Matthew 28:19–20).

However, if you've come to this book with a zeal for God that is already burning white-hot, then keep running hard after Him. My prayer is that this book will be oxygen fanning the flame.

What fire has God set in your life? What is He stirring up in your heart? My heartfelt prayer is that each of God's children will burn bright with zeal for their Father's honor and glory. That akin to fire, this zeal will soften, refine, and purify us as gold. Then, transformed more into His likeness, hearts of stone may become hearts of flesh as they are drawn toward the light of His love radiating from us (see Ezekiel 11:19, 36:26; John 13:35). That our lives may truly count for something and be used for significance by the God who created us.

As the quote at the beginning of the chapter states, "Each of our lives is like an instrument that only God can teach us how to play." May the God-exalting music from our Christ-centered lives become a sacred means whereby the poor, broken, hurting, downtrodden, hopeless, and those who have no idea how much God loves them come to hear the Good News and, perhaps, be healed. You see, it is through the cross-centered lives of more and more of the redeemed—more of God's children seeking His glory and His fame—that the knowledge of His infinite magnificence and unparalleled beauty will progressively cover the earth as the waters cover the sea (see Habakkuk 2:14).

CHAPTER 6

....

A SPARK OF DESIRE

It only takes a spark to get a fire going;
And soon all those around can warm up in its glowing;
That's how it is with God's love, once you've experienced it . . .
You want to sing, it's fresh like spring, you want to pass it on.
—"Pass It On," by Kurt Kaiser

ALTAR OF SACRIFICE

My passion for God began back in 2001. My family had moved from New Jersey to Virginia to be closer to my mother, whose health was declining. When we were looking for a house, I remember telling my husband—half-jokingly, half-seriously—that I didn't want to have to clean up the mess left by someone else. In other words, I really wanted to live in a brand-new house.

Fast-forward three years. After a season of God mercifully pursuing and humbling both my husband and me, the persistent voice of wisdom had gotten louder and louder, drowning out the voice of our own self-centered thinking. God had finally brought us to a place where we clearly understood that the only plans that truly work are

His plans, not ours. As a result of this shift in our understanding, we desired to truly submit to God, to make Him first and foremost in our hearts, and to yield all our plans and desires to Him so that we might single-mindedly pursue His direction.

So my husband and I fervently prayed to be broken of ourselves (see Psalm 51:17)—that God would do whatever He needed to do in our hearts and lives to conform us to Christ. No matter the sacrifice, no matter the inconvenience, no matter how humbling or painful, no matter what the cost, we were ready. My husband had joked that he'd even break-dance in the middle of Bangladesh if God wanted him to.

During this time, we figuratively placed all that God had entrusted to us on the altar. We had also come to recognize that all we had—including ourselves—belonged to God as taught in 1 Corinthians 6:19–20: "Or do you not know that your body is a temple of the Holy Spirit within you, whom you have from God? You are not your own, for you were bought with a price . . ." With mostly glad hearts, we invited God to do anything He wanted with what was His to begin with. We were willing to do without and give up anything that God decided to take away. It slowly dawned on me that by placing everything on the altar, our very lives constituted part of this sacrifice. Undoubtedly, this was the portion of the sacrifice most pleasing to God, for He takes great delight in the offering of a surrendered heart. The fragrance of a heart abandoned to His will is a most sweet aroma wafting up to Heaven.

By grace we continued to seek the Lord, and He instructed us by His Spirit. We came to embrace that obedience is integral to following Christ. We quickly learned that OBEDIENCE has die (to self) right smack in the middle. Pursuing holiness and obeying Jesus were not optional (see 2 Peter 1:3, 5–7; 2 Peter 3:14, 17–18). Having placed ourselves on the sacrificial altar, we soon discovered that the burning off of our sinful ways and familiar habits is a long, painful process.

THIS IS SHELTER?

As it turned out, my darling husband had given in to my desire for a new home. More accurately, I had unwittingly twisted his arm. I vividly recalled him asking me as we signed the sales contract, "Honey, how did we go from looking at homes priced in the upper two hundred thousands to one that's almost half a million dollars?" Now three years later, I had become convicted by Paul's teachings that "But godliness with contentment is great gain, for we brought nothing into the world, and we cannot take anything out of the world. But if we have food and clothing, with these we will be content" (1 Timothy 6:6–8). I remember my shock in realizing that the provision of shelter—which I had previously thought of as one of the most basic needs—is nowhere mentioned in this verse.

Truth be told, this home wasn't really a shelter. Situated in a cul-de-sac on almost three acres of land, we were living in a luxurious mansion compared to more than 99 percent of the world's population. It was a gorgeous 4,300-square-foot home, complete with a stunningly beautiful gourmet kitchen, five bedrooms, a sunroom, an intercom system throughout, a finished basement, and a babbling brook running through the rear of the property. Sure, we needed a house, but in actuality, we had far more house than our family came close to needing. God used this sobering awareness—that our wants are far different from our needs—to do a deeper work in our hearts. His desire to change those who invite Him is relentless, so He took us at our word about being surrendered.

Incidentally, right about this time, the company my husband worked for went under and soon after, he lost his six-figure income. He was given a three-month compensation package, but with the potential downturn in our finances looming, we now stood at a crossroad. My husband could continue working as a computer software developer with a different company—which would have allowed us to maintain our current standard of living—or he could walk away from this career path to pursue what we now knew was God's call on his life: to become a teacher. By God's grace, we resolved to remain steadfast in the center of His will.

But that didn't alleviate our struggles—it compounded them. Shortly after, we found ourselves in serious financial turmoil. My husband concentrated on a business venture he had started just before losing his job, but it failed to be the financial bridge we had hoped. We ended up having to dip into our 401(k) funds.

Admittedly, our first-world challenges didn't come close to third-world challenges, so I'm not equating our experience to the ongoing dire and hopeless situations others have faced. However, after a period of many months, our severe financial difficulties led to some significant hardships. It became a struggle just to provide for the most basic of necessities. We went without heat in the dead of winter for an entire month because we owed $1,000 to the propane company. Dressed in bathrobes whenever in the house, we congregated together next to one of two portable heaters we could afford to keep ourselves warm. For several months, tuna fish sandwiches were a lunch staple, while something as commonplace as eating pizza for dinner became an extravagant luxury we simply couldn't afford.

Nevertheless, we were determined to trust God for all our needs, and He was faithful to provide. At times, He intervened miraculously, like when the propane truck showed up unannounced and completely refilled the propane tank, or when the folks involved in a ministry that my husband had started gave us an unexpected love offering totaling close to $900. This money came at just the right time—when we had absolutely no idea how we'd make the car payment, buy food that week, or put gas in the vehicle for my husband to get to and from his business appointments.

LETTING GO

Although we knew things couldn't continue as they were, we knew even more surely that we wouldn't ignore God's will for my husband to pursue teaching. We sensed God leading us to sell "our" home (possessions and everything God has entrusted to us placed in quotes from here on to denote that nothing we have is really ours)—and He caused that desire to grow. With each passing day, this lovely home lost more and more of its appeal as God enabled me to become increasingly detached from it.

The shift from desiring a brand-new house to no longer being enamored with the house was nothing short of a miracle. My fervent prayer became *Lord, I don't care about this house and I don't want to care about all the other material or temporal things of this world that will someday be destroyed. I just want more and more of You—more of Your presence and Your power in my life!* I started to increasingly resonate with the following line from the hymn "Turn Your Eyes upon Jesus": "Turn your eyes upon Jesus, look full in His wonderful face, and the things of earth will grow strangely dim in the light of His glory and grace."

We put the house on the market, and, praise God, the enemy never succeeded at tempting us to explore opportunities that might have potentially allowed us to keep it. Rather, our primary focus and goal was simply to make the requisite mortgage payments to avert foreclosure. God was gracious and good. Though we came precariously close several times, the house did not go into foreclosure. By this time, we had exhausted a significant portion of "our" 401(k) funds.

During this challenging time, I confessed that not only was I to blame for me and my husband being poor stewards, I had also made the desire for a new home an idol. Since I had been so enamored with the house, I knew deep down that I needed to be completely severed from it. Otherwise, it might have continued to be a snare. In essence,

I knew I needed to fully embrace Mark 9:47: "If your eye causes you to sin, tear it out."

I was very glad when the house did sell and for a very good price—by God's providence we had purchased it when the housing market was low and sold it at its height. With the proceeds from the sale, we liquidated all of our consumer debt. God truly has a great sense of humor. Freedom from financial debt was one of the main reasons that my husband and I had started several business ventures early in our marriage. However, we hadn't fully sought God's guidance with any of them. Now, we had finally realized our dream of being debt-free, albeit not at all like how we had envisioned or could have ever anticipated.

SWEETEST OF TIMES!

So with this wondrous freedom from financial bondage and the trappings of success, God blessed us with a fresh start, fully seeking His direction. He had chastened us out of His fatherly love, but He had also helped us to fix our hearts on Him. Although we went through a very difficult and challenging time, it was yet the sweetest of times. My family and I didn't just come to know God better, we were blessed to have experienced His fatherly care in so many tender and amazing ways.

Many, including Christians, could not understand why we'd sell a beautiful home and downsize. In fact, people often ridicule or criticize those who forsake worldly possessions to wholeheartedly follow after Christ (see Matthew 10:38). Both in and outside the church, many saw our desire to sell out for Christ as plain foolish. Even a few sincere and well-meaning family and friends thought we had gone crazy by selling the house, relinquishing a six-figure income, and throwing away the "success" that we had worked so hard to attain.

We had forsaken the lifestyle we had been accustomed to in order to follow God, and we didn't have many people on our side. Now, we would have to really trust God not only for shelter (as our stellar credit rating had all but plummeted) but also to feed and clothe the three young children He had entrusted to us. God was not limited by our credit rating or any of our circumstances. Indeed, He can do anything but fail! Through a string of divinely orchestrated incidents, He intervened on our behalf and provided us with a three-bedroom town-home. During this new season, we needed to make many sacrifices and adjustments just to *try* to make ends meet. God continued to bless my family—and indeed continues to bless us—in ways beyond what we could have ever imagined. Time after time, God has miraculously shown Himself strong on our behalf.

"Our" children also had to make huge adjustments, but I'm so thankful that my husband and I have given them the opportunity to personally experience what it means to deny oneself and follow Christ. By God's grace, we have demonstrated for them how to not only be detached from the things of this world but also seek first God's kingdom (see Matthew 6:33). We have never once regretted this decision to turn away from pleasing ourselves and to be wholly committed slaves to Christ. While many followers of Christ squirm at the idea of being a "slave" because of what the word connotes, Paul used this vivid imagery to strongly emphasize that we no longer live for our own will but for Christ's instead (see Romans 1:1–15; 1 Corinthians 7:22).

This time of desiring wholehearted surrender to God resulted in a season of tremendous spiritual growth. It also marked the genesis of the deepest and most transformative personal revival that I've ever experienced. In fact, it was in the aftermath of this revival that God ignited in me the spark of desire to follow hard after Him (see Psalm 63:8). I now recognize that without this God-induced brokenness and submission, I could never have come to a place where I earnestly desired to honor God with my life. Truly, without a heart posture of surrender there can be no zeal to live backward for God's glory and fame.

CHAPTER 7
....
THROUGH THE DESERT TO THE HEART OF GOD

To have found God and still to pursue Him is
the soul's paradox of love.
—A. W. Tozer

COMING FOR TOKENS OF LOVE OR JUST OUT OF LOVE

Throughout this season of tremendous spiritual growth, God not only continually drew me to Him, He also empowered me to respond to His displays of love. Often, the cultivation of my relationship with Him didn't happen the way I wanted. Sometimes God took me through wilderness experiences where it felt as though He was playing hide-and-seek with me. I sought Him yet didn't seem to find Him. I say *seem* because, regardless of how we may feel at any point in time, God has promised to never leave us (see Psalm 139:7). There is absolutely nowhere we can run to or hide where God can't bathe us in His grace and wrap us in His love.

Later, I came to understand that God allowed these times to help me avoid a common, self-absorbed preoccupation—seeking emotional highs from our encounters with God. This grieves God. Yet there was a period of time when I was often guilty of this self-centered motive.

Of course God desires us to seek Him and to find joy and satisfaction in His presence. After all, Psalm 16:11 states, "You make known to me the path of life; in your presence there is fullness of joy; at your right hand are pleasures forevermore." It would be seriously wrong if we did not come to God expecting to be satisfied or filled. In fact, as we approach God, we must always see ourselves as needy, and Him as all-sufficient to meet those needs. God also wants us to encounter His presence, for that is when we are changed—when we see His indescribable beauty and holiness, we can't help but apprehend our spiritual poverty and desperate need of Him, which then fuels our desire to be more like Him. But we tend to seek God only for His gifts or for some perceptible awareness of His presence, rather than to fellowship with Him and to truly know Him. God may graciously allow us times when we do experience a sweet or heightened experience of His love or presence. He loves to show up in tangible ways because He delights in ravishing us with His love, filling us with wonder, and doing incredible, even miraculous things, in our midst. But He doesn't always grant this emotional gratification so that we learn to seek Him regardless of whether He chooses to give us a keen sense of His presence. That is always His divine prerogative, not ours. When I didn't understand this spiritual dynamic, I found myself becoming frustrated and disillusioned as I sought after God but didn't "find" Him.

TRANSITIONING FROM MILK TO SOLID FOOD

Spiritual growth and maturity mirrors our physical growth. As we physically grow from infancy to toddlerhood, our diet changes. Which earthly parent, for example, continues to give a four-year-old only a bottle of milk for lunch? Similarly, there eventually comes a time when it would undermine our spiritual growth if God continued to give us milk when we are ready for solid food.

By the same token, a parent may initially reward a child for exhibiting a desired behavior. Eventually, the parent expects the child to internalize the expectation and behave appropriately out of sheer obedience, not just to receive a reward. Likewise, God will not continually reward His children with tokens of His love just because they have responded to Him. Eventually, He, too, desires us to respond out of obedience or the longing to please Him. He wants us to gladly spend time with Him because we simply desire to be in His presence, not just to selfishly experience an emotional high.

We see the same dynamic in human relationships. If a husband only wished to spend time with his wife just to satisfy his own needs and desires, he'd be falling far short of expressing genuine love for her. This is a one-way relationship instead of one that is mutually satisfying and rewarding. The same is true in our relationship with God: we act selfishly if we come to Him only to satisfy our own desires and never attempt to discover, understand, or consider His desires for us.

Here's an encouraging way to look at this spiritual reality: you can be certain you're turning your eyes away from yourself and focusing more on God when you seek fellowship with Him even though He has stopped giving you emotional highs. It means you're growing spiritually as your requirements are becoming less self-centered and more God-centered. The beautiful irony is that the more we fix our gaze upon God, the more He floods our hearts, souls, and minds with greater revelations of Himself—in ways far deeper and more solid than emotional highs. Abandoning our self-seeking requests to truly know God's heart is a sincere expression of surrender, and this greatly pleases our Father.

As we delight God's heart, He delights ours. It's like God gives us back what we have freely given Him, except what He gives back is far greater than what we've given Him. He delights to pour out blessing after blessing on those who continually seek to dethrone the self and enthrone Christ in their hearts. Yet we must always remain mindful that blessings come to us only through the righteousness of Christ (see 2 Corinthians 5:21); we do not earn them because we are in any way deserving.

I also know from experience that when we seek God but don't experience an emotional high, we're tempted to seek Him less diligently or to stop seeking Him altogether. Generally, the longer we postpone doing something that we need to do, the harder it becomes to rouse the motivation to do it. So the longer we go without spending time with God, the harder it is to get back in the habit of seeking Him again. I want to encourage you to keep pressing on, even if you're currently devoting only a brief period of time to Him. In the long run, it's far easier to gradually increase the time we spend with God—and still experience growth, albeit more slowly—than it is to start all over once we've neglected pursuing intimacy with God for a long period of time. Beware of the schemes of the enemy who is not only fully aware of this natural human tendency but also exploits it, to our great detriment.

DEVELOPING INTIMACY

In hindsight, what helped me persevere through the dry times— when I was more focused on my emotional desires than seeking true connection with God—was this reassurance: "You will seek me and find me, when you seek me with all your heart" (Jeremiah 29:13). I eventually discovered that seeking God had nothing at all to do with getting what my little heart wanted. Rather, it meant humbly coming to God in brokenness: praising Him, thanking Him, petitioning Him in accordance to His will, seeking to be like Him, confessing and repenting of my sins, and so on. My faithfulness in pursuing God was also bolstered by James 4:8: "Draw near to God, and he will draw near to you."

As I look back, I clearly see that God enabled me to draw near to Him by taking away those emotional experiences that I so badly wanted. He began by continually reminding me that He knew what was best for me. Then He challenged me to come to Him expecting to receive only what He wanted to give me. This meant trusting Him to give me just what I needed, not necessarily what I wanted. Coming to Him without preconceived expectations progressively became easier and easier. I'm so thankful that God is such a wise, loving, and judicious Father. I'm grateful that He didn't give me milk when I needed solid food, and that He waited patiently for me to disassociate my pursuit of Him from receiving tokens of His love.

As it turns out, the dry times I had experienced did not lessen my hunger for God. God instead used those times to deepen my hunger and thirst for Him. The more I didn't seem to find Him, the more determined I became. Persistence paid off. Eventually, God gave me the desire to study and pore over His Word in order to know Him more intimately. I came to understand that knowing God and knowing about God are two entirely different things; many learned, dedicated scholars of the Bible have extensive knowledge of God yet do not know God. Similarly, many self-professed followers know of Christ but don't really know Him. Intimacy changes that.

STEPPING ON THE HEELS OF JESUS

Later, I came to discover that whenever God took me through dry and barren seasons, it was just a matter of time before He'd bring me to yet another oasis of truth—a place where He'd open the eyes of my heart and allow me to glimpse more of His attributes and character. These wilderness times always led me into the Promised Land, where sweet encounters with God were nourishing and soothing to my soul. It was this anticipation of spiritual refreshment that sustained me during those sometimes long and difficult seasons. Seasons, for example, when I wanted to be following Jesus so closely that I almost stepped on His heels but instead felt like I was lagging so very far behind Him. I was thrilled to discover that the very fact I was hungry for more of God was in and of itself a guarantee that I would be satisfied. Why? Because God revealed His promise, "Blessed are those who hunger and thirst for righteousness, for they *shall* be satisfied" (Matthew 5:6; emphasis mine). Time and again, this promise reenergized my earnest pursuit of Him.

STOPPING THE WORLD FOR ME?

Contrasting the dry times, there were periods when God overwhelmed me with tender displays of His love. I learned that God was not only capable of relating to me in uniquely personal ways but also that He wants to and longs to. At various times, God has orchestrated multiple activities in my sphere just to show me how much He loves me—like when He seemed to pull out all the stops to ensure that a complicated application involving several different parties that should have taken several weeks to get processed was somehow completed in just a few days. God knew the urgency of the situation and sovereignly worked on my behalf to make what seemed impossible possible.

At other times, God has provided for a specific personal need behind the scenes. I'll always remember the day many years ago when I just had a feeling that I needed to go visit my mother. While driving there, I was praying and asking God to make a way for us to purchase a much-needed vacuum cleaner. After I had visited with my mother, I prepared to leave. Just before I headed out, my brother showed up unexpectedly and we chatted for a few minutes. After I gave him a hug good-bye, he gently took my right hand and slipped something into it. When I opened my hand, I couldn't believe my eyes. My dear brother had given me a crisp hundred-dollar bill, something he had never done before. I had only some of the money for the new vacuum and had prayed on the way to my mother's that God would graciously provide the balance. I had eighty-nine in the bank, and the vacuum cleaner that

I wanted was exactly $189! My brother had no idea about any of this. Truly, we serve a good and awesome God who attentively cares for His children!

When God is in the process of drawing our hearts nearer to Him, He often woos us by blessing us with concrete displays of His love, as he did for me in the two above examples. As I reflect on my life, I realize that God's special tokens of love toward me were consistent with Romans 2:4: "God's kindness is meant to lead you to repentance." With certainty, God's goodness and kindness toward me fueled my desire to love Him more deeply and to forsake my will for His. The more God revealed how much He loved me, the more I wanted to love Him in return. More and more, I wanted to please Him by the way I lived; I desperately wanted Christ to be magnified in my life. So much so that I sometimes desired to be supersanctified in a figurative blaze of glory and have huge chunks of my sinful thought patterns and behaviors burned off at one time. (Note: For clarity, I use sanctification here in the sense of being progressively transformed by the truth of God's Word [see 2 Corinthians 3:18; 1 Thessalonians 4:3], not in the other sense of God having already sanctified us by justification through our faith in Christ [see Acts 26:18; 1 Corinthians 1:2, 6:11].)

My naïve expectation made the sanctification process seem all the slower. I've now learned that sanctification rarely goes as fast as we may like, for the simple reason that we are stubborn and self-absorbed. It takes much time to be broken of our sinful tendencies. Indeed, the sanctification process is analogous to cooking with a slow Crock-Pot, not the microwave as we might prefer. Nevertheless, throughout this time, I remained ever grateful that God was not only drawing me to Him but also giving me the desire to come. I also came to grasp God's extravagant love for His children, as well as His passionate desire for them to single-mindedly pursue Him. To say an ardent pursuit of God is more than worth it is truly one of the greatest understatements we could ever make—as we've previously mentioned, truly nothing and no one else can satisfy our intense longings or fulfill the deepest desires of our hearts.

GOD: EVER-PURSUING, EVER-CHASING

My ever-increasing desire to honor God with my life was proof of His persistent yet inscrutable workmanship on my heart. I knew well that my desire to seek God was not the result of my own willingness or self-effort. In fact, despite all the times that I continued to give in to my sinful desires, God continued to steadfastly pursue me. He was zealous for an intimate relationship with me and wanted me to have the same yearning for Him.

Then came my discovery of an amazing, reciprocal loop! I realized that the more I sought God, the more I found Him. The more I found Him, the more I knew Him. And the more I knew Him, the more I couldn't help but love Him more! I also discovered that when we look for God's hand—His mercy, patience, goodness, and faithfulness—as we go about everyday life, we find it. Each time we glimpse God's activity in our lives, we're reminded of His constant love and care. It was seeing God's intimate involvement in my life over time that essentially enabled me to become completely overwhelmed by His love for me as an individual person. The more I understood just how much it cost God to make me a recipient of His extravagant love, the more I wanted to worship and adore Him; the more I treasured Him, the more I wanted to live for His glory. All along, He had been wooing me into an intimate relationship with Him, one wherein I would gladly embrace the words of Christ, "My food is to do the will of him who sent me" (John 4:34).

Having wooed me and brought me to a place of wholehearted submission, God had had His say and captured my heart; He had subdued my stubborn will—and although I stumbled time and time again, I now no longer desired to gratify my flesh. When my self-will tried to assert itself, the Holy Spirit would remind me that this was contrary to His desires. For example, when I would become angry by how someone had treated me and wanted to hold a grudge or act in spite, He reminded me that love is patient and kind, not irritable or resentful (see 1 Corinthians 13:4–8). He progressively empowered me to not give in to my desires. In denying myself more, I grieved Him less.

God had supernaturally rescued me from being a slave to my self-love, a love that was quite strong and robust. After all, I had taken the utmost care to nurture and appease it for well over three decades! For instance, through the years, many long, late-night discussions that ensued between my husband and me were the result of my being overly focused on myself—what I thought I wanted or needed that he had failed to provide. After chatting at length and hearing his side, I'd often realize that the entire conversation had been a waste of valuable time and emotional energy, not to mention the loss of sleep. Were it not for my self-love, most of those arguments could have and would have been avoided. I've since learned that nothing good or worthy ever comes out of a preoccupation with one's self. God also enabled me to clearly see the steep price that my self-love was costing me: it had been (and for quite some time after continued to be) the seedbed of most of my misery, heartaches, and disappointments in my life. So not only for God's glory but also for my own good—my emotional well-being, the leadership of His Spirit in my life, my spiritual growth, "my" marriage, "my" nuclear family—I was glad that God, not self, had become uppermost in my heart. Now more than ever, I wanted my attitude and conduct to bring joy to my Father's heart and keep a smile on His face.

I BECAME A BEGGAR

God had offered me the gift of desiring to follow hard after Him. By His mysterious inner workings, I had accepted it! This acceptance then transformed me into a consummate beggar. Among other heartfelt requests, I begged God for wisdom. I pleaded with Him to help me increasingly sense the leading of His Spirit. I implored Him to remove my cravings for the artificially sweetened things of this world that have no lasting value that I may progressively taste and see that the Lord is good (see Psalm 34:8). I prayed with desperation for God to show me the wonderful truths in His Word that I may "run in the way of [His] commandments" (Psalm 119:32). I sincerely wanted to say with Job, "I have treasured the words of his mouth more than my portion of food" (Job 23:12). I longed to join my voice with David's exclamation: "How sweet are your words to my taste, sweeter than honey to my mouth!" (Psalm 119:103).

In short, I begged God to help me truly become His living temple (see 2 Corinthians 6:16), to empower me to live a life that continually imaged forth more of His glory. In response, He gave me a seemingly unquenchable thirst to know Him better and to love Him more. I was able to sincerely say, "As a deer pants for flowing streams, so pants my soul for you, O God" (Psalm 42:1). God graciously met me as I sought Him, and the precious times experienced in His presence enabled me to identify with the words: "For a day in your courts is better than a thousand elsewhere" (Psalm 84:10). That spark of desire He had ignited in me had undeniably turned into a flame.

What I've shared in this chapter is the process whereby God set ablaze in my heart a zeal to honor Him with how I live. My "life verse" became Isaiah 26:8–9 (New Living Translation): "Lord, we show our trust in you by obeying your laws; *our heart's desire is to glorify your name.* In the night I search for you; in the morning I earnestly seek you" (emphasis mine). It seemed that all the desires God had ever so patiently wrought in me could be distilled into this one passage of Scripture.

CHAPTER 8
....
CULINARY CREATIONS

For we are the aroma of Christ to God among those who
are being saved and among those who are perishing.
—2 Corinthians 2:15

THE MASTER CHEF

I've discussed how God gave me a passion to seek after Him and how
it played out in my life, ultimately stimulating in me the desire to live
for His renown. But this is only half of the story. I believe it's also
important to not only give some insights into what I was like prior to
this change but also explain what God's work in our hearts really looks
like so we know what we can expect as we move forward in building a
truly significant life.

In so doing, I liken God's workmanship in my life to being graciously invited into His divine kitchen—a most instrumental place in
preparing us to live backward. God has taken the truths He's revealed
to me over the past several years and used them as ingredients to display His extraordinary culinary expertise, despite the blandness of my
heart. I look back now and see how God has wondrously changed me

in ways that I myself can hardly believe. Truly, His work of progressive transformation in such a formerly selfish and prideful person as myself has been nothing short of masterful! God's relentless determination to somehow make a tasty culinary dish out of my unappetizing flavor is responsible for the freedom and joy that I have in Christ, the seasoning that permeates my life. This is His desire for you too.

As you might imagine, God's transformation of our hearts resembles anything but a basic cooking class. Charles Spurgeon said, "The sustenance of the whole universe, I do believe, is even less than this— the changing of a bad heart, the subduing of an iron will."[17] Indeed, left to itself, the human heart is corrupt and extremely obstinate. The process of transforming our hearts from being self-centered to God-centered requires divine omniscience and skill, coupled with a complex variety of intricate techniques. Therefore, God is like a master chef at work in our hearts. Similar to modifying a recipe until it reaches perfection, God is ever seeking to purify us because He desires each of His children to become a refined specialty dish. Each dish, of course, is one of His signature classics, composed of its own unique combination of ingredients—some common, as in the weaknesses or flaws that we all experience; some unusual, as in a special gift; others even exotic, as in a rare ability or a very unique calling. Although unlimited in scope, the expert chef's unparalleled methods for transforming each dish are not only highly specialized, they're, of course, also individualized. Mostly indiscernible to our finite minds, they are precisely timed and carefully administered to bring about results aimed at both our greatest good and the display of His glory.

Moreover, the chef thoroughly understands all the varied processes and iterations necessary to continually refine each dish. Since God exists outside of time, He can see, even now, the perfectly finished dishes. For the time being, He is content that each dish is not

---

17. Charles Spurgeon, *The Fullness of Joy* (New Kensington: Whitaker House, 1997), 25.

completely perfect, so long as each continues to take on more of the look, taste, texture, and appeal that He desires.

Quite often we do not take too kindly to the chef's carefully selected methods or processes and thus stubbornly refuse to cooperate. When this occurs, the unsurpassed chef must employ rather intensive techniques in order to keep the cooking process moving along. In other words, the challenges and trials we sometimes experience in life can be the direct result of the chef's concentrated—but always loving—measures to make us more pliable in His hands. For example, I remember when God got my full attention by shattering an idol I had erected yet wasn't even aware of, namely, my marriage. For several months, I was in a state of emotional upheaval. Nevertheless, God lovingly redeemed both the difficult time that ensued and my shortcoming, using both to help me better understand how He desires me to love and honor my husband while still keeping Him uppermost in my life. As a result, our marriage was placed on more solid ground, and our husband and I began to enjoy an even sweeter relationship than we had before experienced.

When we actually consider just how self-willed the dishes instinctively tend to be, it's nothing short of a miracle that the process moves along as well as it does, or that change, however slowly, even occurs. But then again, this is what an expert generally does—he makes the seemingly impossible possible. In this case, the divine expert literally *does* what is impossible for us—He softens our hard, rebellious hearts! How reassuring to know that our hearts, our minds, our understanding, and our continued spiritual growth are always in the hands of the wisest and greatest Expert in the universe.

THE PERFECT BALANCE

And to think that this culinary expert is also our Abba! "Abba" is an Aramaic word that would most closely be translated as "Papa" or

"Daddy." A term of endearment, it signifies the close bond between children and their beloved father, as well as the childlike trust that should characterize this relationship (see John 1:12–13). However, I do want to recognize and be sensitive to those who have never experienced this kind of relationship with their earthly father. Be reassured that standing in Christ, God will never hurt you, abandon you, or fail you as some earthly fathers do; more than you can even begin to imagine, He values you as His child and longs to show you His unending love.

Before going further, I want to digress from the divine kitchen because it's important to understand God's fatherly role in our lives. In disciplining their children, earthly parents often have difficulty striking the right balance between being loving while at the same time remaining firm. However, because our Abba is the only perfectly wise Father, He not only knows how to achieve this flawless balance in the discipline of His children, He is also fully capable of accomplishing it. However, we must recognize that inasmuch as God is perfect in His justice and righteousness, He is also perfect in His love and compassion. God never capriciously chastens His children. Moreover, God's character is unchanging; therefore, we can trust Him to be not one iota tougher than required. Likewise, our Father will not be any less gentle than necessary. He always strikes the effective balance of firmness and love.

We are assured: "the Lord disciplines the one he loves, and chastises every son whom he receives" (Hebrews 12:6; see also Proverbs 13:12; Revelations 3:19). We should actually feel cause for concern if we sense or believe that God is withholding His discipline from us (see Hebrews 12:8). Nevertheless, because our heavenly Father is good, merciful, and all-knowing, He sovereignly orchestrates each and every one of our life circumstances, allowing us to experience only what He knows we need for continued progress—never less and never more.

Indeed, God would be unloving and unwise were He to allow us to endure less than what is required for our continued growth; in the same vein, were God to allow us to suffer unnecessarily, simply for the sake of suffering, it would be cruel of Him and contrary to His holy nature. When I view my need for discipline through the lens of God's love, I am thankful that my Father is continually molding and shaping me to be more like Him. I recognize that any hardships, difficulties, and trials that I experience because of His chastening hand are because He ultimately wishes to bring out the very best in me.

Though imperfectly demonstrated, isn't this the same desire that we see in earthly parents who truly love the children whom God has entrusted to them and want their best? I was blessed to have had wonderful parents like this. But although they were very loving, fair, and did a good job of pointing me toward God, I wasn't exposed to regular biblical discipleship while growing up. I didn't know or understand many of the precepts in God's Word. I was also naïve to many key spiritual realities. There was much that I needed to both learn and unlearn about God as a thirtysomething. It is from within this context that God brought me into His divine kitchen and began His transformative work in my heart.

REFINING THE DISH

We've seen that God exercises the perfect balance of gentleness and firmness with His children because He is determined for us to look more like Him. However, it's critical to emphasize that as God progressively molds us into the image of Christ "that we may share his holiness" (Hebrews 12:10), He will also judiciously spare nothing in His chastisement of us.

As I mentioned earlier, I'm well acquainted with the processes and techniques employed by the divine chef. Allow me to now explain what they have looked like for me. Indeed, they will likely look different for you, as God relates to each of us as unique individuals, each at different places in our spiritual growth and development.

Over the years, God has lovingly revealed my sinful ways to me, gently exposing my wrong beliefs for what they are. He has unveiled my tendency toward legalism, that deeply rooted proclivity to think we merit God's favor by our good works, and exposed my complacency in not doing those things that I know I should. He's taken my judgmental attitude and washed it like a filthy dish cloth and hung it up to dry. As for my hypocrisy, He's put it on full display in the window of my heart. In response to my selfishness, God constantly tells me that it's not about me!

The Holy Spirit also sifted out clumps of errors and chunks of misconceptions from my thoughts and my mind. For example, there was a period in my life when, though I wasn't faultfinding with others, my verbal responses to the children I'm blessed with were often more critical than encouraging. I had not the slightest notion I was even behaving in such a critical manner until the Holy Spirit put a spotlight on this verse: "Let everything you say be good and helpful, so that your words will be an encouragement to those who hear them" (Ephesians 4:29, New Living Translation). I mentally kept track of my comments for two weeks and was both shocked and dismayed at the sheer number of times my words had not been edifying. But by continually meditating on this verse, the Holy Spirit brought me to a place where He'd simply nudge me when I was about to say something critical, enabling me to catch myself before speaking it out. After He helped me to drastically decrease the frequency of my unhelpful remarks, the Holy Spirit did an even deeper work, resulting in fewer critical thoughts in the first place. Finally, He enabled me to cultivate the practice of not saying anything at all if I had nothing positive to say. In the process, God completely shattered my misconception of myself as someone who wasn't at all faultfinding.

God also weighed my motives for *why* I do *what* I do, and, often, they were found grossly misguided. If you've ever committed to something only because you wanted to derive a personal benefit, then you know exactly what I mean. As I began to embrace God's teaching to do nothing out of selfish ambition or vain conceit (see Philippians 2:3–4), God helped me to gradually overcome this natural tendency. He first gave me a deeper desire to have a clean and pure heart before Him (see Psalm 24:4), and then empowered me to prayerfully consider only those things that I believed He was leading me to pursue for His glory.

My self-absorption—often expressed when my restless desire to receive credit for what I had done went unmet—was so chronic that God needed to tenderly beat it out of me at the highest blender speed. He chopped up my pride when He showed me that the reason I was becoming so upset over my failures and shortcomings was not primarily because I had fallen short of His glory, but, rather, because I was seeing myself for who I truly was, and I didn't like what I was seeing. Time and time again, He showed me my prideful tendencies, like when I went back into the house (having already gotten into the car headed to a class) to swap a generic bottle of water with a name brand. Why? Just so that I'd be seen with the Deer Park brand instead. How ridiculous!

He then proceeded to mince into bits my self-reliance, many times causing me to fall flat on my face when I failed to look to Him for strength and guidance. Although I haven't completely overcome the tendency to procrastinate at times, I've made much progress in this area, thanks to God diligently churning it out of me. My lack of integrity— for example, purposefully omitting a detail that doesn't cast me in a positive light when relaying a personal experience—has been diced into pieces, then pounded with a meat tenderizer.

God uses my wrong attitudes, self-driven habits, and sinful tendencies to keep me humbled; they're a continual reminder of how messed up I still am and how desperately I need Christ, moment by moment. Besides promoting humility, choosing to focus on what God still needs to do in my heart guards me from being judgmental and critical of others. This attitude is so important. Following the biblical model, disciples are called to judge or keep one another accountable for walking out holiness and leave those outside the church to God (see 1 Corinthians 5:12–13). However, the first sin that we must each overcome is the innate tendency to judge others, as it clouds our ability to see sin within ourselves (see Matthew 7:4–5; Luke 6:42). As I seek God's help to overcome my shortcomings, I am more willing to extend grace and mercy to others instead of judging them. In other words, I desire to see and focus on the best in people. We hit a major milestone in our spiritual growth when we feel compassion for others, rather than rebuke or criticism.

God doesn't just work on how we treat others or the fruit that we bear; He also works on our interior or thought lives. Since Scripture plays a major part in how God transforms us, He desires that our minds marinate daily in the Bible. God's Word searches out and exposes the sin and corruption still in our hearts. For instance, as my mind is progressively illumined to the truths in God's Word, the impurities in my heart have continued to rise to the surface, where they are skimmed off by the master chef. It is because of this continual renewal of my mind that God has time and again challenged my convictions, tested my attitude, transformed my motives, gently reproved my thoughts and behavior, and realigned my values. Despite messy countertops splattered with a mixture of my constant failures and weaknesses, a ceiling adorned with huge globs of complacency stew, and a kitchen floor soiled by the tracks of besetting sins, much good has come out of all this ruckus and disorder in the divine kitchen of my life.

Although my self-love relentlessly tries to make a comeback, its attempts are squelched more and more by the lordship of Christ—relinquishing control of what I want in favor of what He desires. When my self-love regrettably does get its way, I'm keenly reminded just how far I have yet to go. Overall, because I less frequently sit on the throne of my heart, there are not as many "me and mine" tantrums as before. Thanks to this remarkable coup wrought by the Spirit of God, I'm delighted to say that many of my selfish desires and tendencies have found their way into the garbage disposal. In fact, I actually have come to expect far less from other people in regards to "getting my way."

I CAN SEE BETTER NOW!

The divine kitchen is also intended to give us spiritual eye-openers. For example, there was a time when I thought that the more I pursued holiness, the more I would somehow *see* that I was becoming more like Christ. I've since learned the error in viewing spiritual growth in this way. Although the chef has been using His blender on me for quite some time now, there's still a lot of impurities in my heart and mind. This reality led to an ironic discovery: as the Holy Spirit shows me my self-driven tendencies and patterns of behavior, I better apprehend just how sinful my heart initially was and indeed continues to be, even after all these years of God's relentless refining process. As I cooperate with God to purify my heart, I don't see less of my sinfulness; rather, I see even more clearly just how much I fall short of His glory. It overwhelms me that God continues to work with this messed-up dish. Even more amazing and incredible is that God has already seen me at my worse yet loves me and continues to put up with me.

In addition to the blending, heating, and other methods, He frequently adds flavor-enhancing virtues: stirring in spoonfuls of gentleness, mixing in a pint of love, folding in a cup of compassion, and so on. I really don't know where I'd be without the divine chef's persistent faithfulness and kindness.

Despite my flesh persistently attempting to obstruct the process every step of the way, I've become even more supple and malleable in the chef's masterful hands. God continues to stir in me a deep desire to grow in godliness. Judging by the current state of this dish, I know there's a lot of work still to be done. Thankfully, it is a whole lot better than it used to be.

THE CHEF IS THE "GOODEST"!

What a glorious transformative experience this has been! In general, the kitchen seems to be less messy now. But notice that I say "seems." That's because God's divine kitchen—located in the depths of my heart—is just like the physical kitchen of the current abode God has blessed me with: I just can't seem to keep it sparkling clean for long periods of time. One moment the sink is clean and empty, then almost immediately the children have a snack or make something for lunch, and there goes the sparkling kitchen. My heart's the same way: messy one moment, seemingly clean another. But no matter how clean I may perceive my heart to be at any given moment, my finite, deceitful mind will always conspire to cloud the true condition of my soul. Although I can't know the actual state of my heart, much less see it, God knows and sees it all. Thankfully, we have His indwelling presence to overcome any and all sinful tendencies and to subdue any temptations that we may face (1 Corinthians 10:13).

Without a doubt there are still times when I feel as though the counters and floors in my heart are a royal mess, as the chef diligently works to conform me to Christ: beating and whisking out impure motives and desires, folding and stirring in nuggets of truth, pureeing and grinding sinful tendencies. Truth be told, the messy kitchen is not optional, nor can it be avoided. Christ did not say, "If anyone will come after me, let him pursue his own desires and do whatever he pleases." No. Jesus said, "If anyone will come after me, let him *deny* himself and take up his cross and follow me" (Matthew 16:24). To follow Jesus involves sacrifice, which is neither convenient nor comfortable to our natural feelings and inclinations.

So I want to caution you that when the chef goes to work, there's always going to be a whole lot of mess. Also, the cleanup—the growth, change, and victories—may not come for a long time or as often as we'd like. Nevertheless, our chef is good—very, very good! In fact,

He is what I've coined, the "goodest." And as I've mentioned, He does all things marvelously well! Because of His skillful workmanship and promise to complete the good work that He has already begun in us, we have every reason to trust and believe that we will become better still and indeed come to completion (see Philippians 1:6). So stick with His masterful culinary process in your own life. I assure you, you will not be disappointed. In fact, you too will stand back and marvel at what He has wrought in you.

Yet I don't want to minimize the fact that this process can be very difficult. While you may recognize that the refining is necessary, you may be feeling as though you can't take the heat of the kitchen much longer. Understandable, but be encouraged; remember that our Father's state-of-the-divine appliances will not be used on you one moment longer than is absolutely necessary. So don't despair of God's inner workings in your life and don't try to avoid critical steps in the process. Otherwise, you will proverbially jump from the frying pan into the fire itself, where the heat is even more intense. Instead, ask God to help you endure His expert simmering, sautéing, or whatever process He deems necessary so that He may accomplish in you what He desires and so that you don't forfeit valuable lessons and undermine your growth in Christ. It *is* hard, but remember that we have all the grace and help we need through the indwelling presence and power of the Holy Spirit.

FIT FOR THE KING OF KINGS

God will indeed transform each of His children into a perfectly seasoned and refined culinary creation. One glorious day, at the future wedding feast of the King of Kings, He will unveil His exquisite culinary dishes (see Revelations 19:6–9). The marriage banquet of Christ and His Bride have been in the works since before even the foundations of the earth were set! Can you even begin to imagine what this divine celebration will be like? Or what it will be like to be completely free of sin? God Himself will present each of us—His vessels of honor—blameless before the presence of his glory and with exceedingly great joy (see Jude 24). I don't know about you, but on that glorious day, I deeply desire to be a beautiful and polished vessel with whom my heavenly Father is well pleased. Until then, I want to be ever soft and supple in the chef's hands so that He may accomplish in my life all that He desires.

God graciously invites each of His children into this culinary process and into His divine kitchen, where He lovingly prepares our hearts. It does involve beating and whisking, pounding and heating, but along the way are taste tests—God-ordained opportunities where we must choose in the moment to not react in a fleshly manner but respond in a Christlike way—which accurately determine whether the dishes are becoming more savory to our Father in Heaven and, thus, seasoned just enough to influence the world for Christ.

Are you that refined dish in which God sees Himself glorified in such a way that He wants to unveil you to the world? Perhaps! Meanwhile, may the master chef continue His prepping and cooking—sanctifying, purifying, and refining our hearts so that the world may notice that our lives are robustly seasoned with the Spirit of Christ. Scripture teaches, "For we are the aroma of Christ to God among those who are being saved and among those who are perishing, to one a fragrance from death to death, to the other a fragrance from life to life" (2 Corinthians 2:15). May the fragrant aroma of our Christ-centered lives waft into and penetrate the air, taking God's glory and renown wherever we may go, even to the farthest corners of the earth. I want to encourage and challenge you to wholeheartedly embrace this culinary process, for the praise of God's great glory and, of course, your immeasurable gain.

PRINCIPLE 2

CULTIVATE A PASSIONATE LOVE FOR GOD

CHAPTER 9

ADOPTION INTO GOD'S FAMILY

See what kind of love the Father has given to
us, that we should be called children of God.
—1 John 3:1

ANCESTRY 101

In the previous chapter, I shared various aspects of my flaws and shortcomings, as well as God's dealings in my heart. I also discussed that as my understanding of God's fatherly love has deepened, so has my desire to be more like Him and to please Him. I've discovered that integral to living backward is becoming awestruck by our Father's extravagant love for us—what it is, how it was effected, and what it means.

The result of Adam and Eve's disobedience to God in the Garden is that each of us is born with a fallen or sinful nature (see Genesis 3). But I sometimes hear people say that we shouldn't be held accountable for the sin committed by Adam and Eve. So I think it's important to quickly address this concern before going any further.

Romans 5:19 says of Adam: "by the one man's disobedience the many were made sinners." This means that, fundamentally, we all are born sinners because Adam disobeyed God. Our behavior and the sins we commit are secondary to the fact that we were born into a family apart from God. So by virtue of simply being Adam's descendants, his disobedience and sin has been passed on to us. Because of this inherited sin, not a single one of us can approach God on our own merit. This biblical truth removes any grounds for a person to argue that he or she is a "good" person and can thus claim righteousness before God on the basis of "goodness" (see Psalm 53:1; Ecclesiastes 7:20; Romans 3:10–12). If someone isn't prepared to fully accept this truth, he or she must also be willing to forfeit the promise that goes along with Adam's disobedience. It is found in the second half of Romans 5:19: "so by [Jesus's] obedience the many will be made righteous" (see also 1 Corinthians 15:21–22).

This means that the problem of sin is far deeper than how each of us behaves. The Bible does not refer to us as sinners primarily because we commit sins; on the contrary, we sin because we are sinners in our fallen state or out of fellowship with God. In fact, our natural proclivity to sin is undeniable evidence that we are born with sinful natures. This is why no one ever has to teach a two-year-old to shout "Mine!" or a four-year-old to lie about sneaking a cookie from the cookie jar. This understanding of how we came to be sinners and our personal responsibility for our sins is critical.

DOUBLY IN NEED OF GRACE

Whether or not we are aware of it, the sin and evil in our hearts place us in desperate, desperate need of God. However, these same sinful hearts also make it impossible for us to ever come to God of our own accord or desire. God hates sin because it is contrary to His holy and perfect nature (see Isaiah 6:3). As sinners, therefore, we are utterly separated from God (see Isaiah 59:2). The Bible goes so far as to say that, outside of a relationship with God, we are actually objects of His wrath, consigned to everlasting condemnation because the wages of our sin is death—both physical and spiritual (see Romans 3:9). Not only are we separated from God, our sinful condition also renders us incapable of ever seeking Him (see Psalm 14:1–3; Romans 3:11). Left to ourselves, all of us are completely unwilling to come to God. Scripture teaches that no sinner can make the choice to come to God on his own because each of us is unable to understand, to repent, and to believe (see Jeremiah 31:3; John 6:44–45, 65; Romans 3:10–12). In theology, this is referred to as prevenient grace: before a person can draw near to God, God must first have drawn the person to Himself. Absent of God's infinite grace and mercies, there would unequivocally be no remedy for our fatal sin disease. Thus, we could say that we are *doubly* in need of God's grace to save us.

We need to really grasp this: absolutely nothing in our fallen nature desires God. This is because our hearts are hardened and unregenerate— not only do we commit sins, we are also sinful to our very core (see Genesis 8:21; Jeremiah 17:9; Psalm 51:5; Ephesians 2:1–3). Because we actually enjoy the pleasures of sin, we have no inherent desire to stop sinning (see John 3:20–21). As a result, we are hostile toward God; the very nature of sin is akin to shaking one's fist and vehemently shouting, "God, I don't need you!" Sin makes us refuse to seek a cure for our terminal disease because we refuse to admit we even have one.

To sin is to transgress against the holiness of God, to offend God, violate His Word, and fall short of His glory. In seeking to gratify ourselves, we fail to place supremacy on the inestimable worth of God's glory—we exalt ourselves over God. This outright rebellion, besides cutting us off from God, also undergirds our false sense of self-sufficiency. In so doing, sin blinds us to God's truth and the reality of our actions. That's why we cannot eventually come to our senses and decide to seek God. He must seek us first.

RAISING THE DEAD, PHYSICALLY AND SPIRITUALLY

Ever heard the story of Lazarus? Jesus called him forth from the grave after he had been dead for almost three days. But until Jesus spoke the words of life that summoned Lazarus's decaying body from the tomb, he was completely incapable of helping himself. This is a picture of our helplessness—blinded by sin, we too are utterly powerless to respond to God's call, much less submit to His laws (see Romans 8:7). Not only are we blinded by sin but also we are dead in our sins (see Romans 3:23), unable to do anything to help ourselves.

Like Lazarus, we all are like corpses without God. Since we are lifeless, God must regenerate us or awaken us from spiritual death before we can positively respond to His call. The good news is that the Gospel raises dead men back to life. Something truly radical occurs. God first regenerates our hearts. He replaces a heart of stone with a heart of flesh—a heart that desires to seek Him (see Ezekiel 11:19). This is referred to as new birth. As a result of this supernatural experience, we receive a life that we did not possess before—an altogether new and divine life.

Thus, regeneration is a gift God gives us, because it can only be initiated or induced by Him. But regeneration is more than a gift. It is nothing short of a miracle because it makes possible that which is absolutely impossible for man (see Luke 18:27). Blind eyes see, deaf ears hear, and a hardened heart is made soft.

PICTURE OF PERFECT SURRENDER

The story didn't begin with God having to bring dead men back to life. I want to encourage those familiar with the salvation story to read it below as if it were new, allowing its awesome truths to fill you with joy, wonder, and deep gratitude.

Adam and Eve enjoyed complete harmony, fellowship, and intimacy with God—until they disobeyed God. At that moment both physical and spiritual death entered the world, creating a chasm that completely separated man from God. This is the utterly hopeless condition that every human is born into. We are destined to partake of the blazing anger and consuming wrath of a holy God for all of eternity.

But God in His rich mercy always had a plan to circumvent our ancestors' decision to disobey Him. Beyond the limits of what we can fully understand, the all-powerful Son of God would surrender His will and come into the earth that He created as fully man, without relinquishing his deity. As fully God and fully man, He would then be capable of leading a perfectly holy and surrendered life on the earth precisely because, as fully God, He was incapable of sin. By virtue of His holy and sinless life, Jesus would essentially become the perfect sacrificial Lamb—He would once and for all put an end to the imperfect Old Testament sacrificial system that God Himself had established for His people (the Israelites) to make amends for their sins (see Exodus 12:3, 6; Leviticus 4:2, 17:11; 1 Peter 1:19–20). Essentially, Jesus would take the place of guilty sinners and incur all of His Father's consuming wrath against sin in order to satisfy the demands of His Father's justice against sin (see Isaiah 53:12). In so doing, He would exchange His divine perfection for the repulsiveness of our sins so that we, in turn, could trade all our sins for His divine perfection. As a result of this inconceivable transaction—this unfathomable price of redemption— Jesus Christ would become the solution to our unsolvable sin problem, reconciling us back to God (see Romans 5:10).

TRADING THE GLORIES OF HEAVEN FOR DISHONOR

God's eternal plan became reality. Jesus came into the world as a human. Born of His virgin mother, Mary, in a nondescript manger, the Lord of the universe and King of Majesty became a helpless babe. As is the natural growth process for any child, He was a boy who subsequently became a man. (Can you picture him throwing rocks, playing with dirt, and climbing trees?) Yet he never sinned. On the contrary, Jesus learned obedience in the earth by being perfectly submitted to His Father in Heaven. In fact, carrying out His Father's will was the driving force and ruling passion of his life here on earth.

In preparation for His earthly ministry, Jesus was led into the wilderness by the devil, where, in addition to being tempted, he went without food and water for forty days. But this was just the beginning. Jesus was scorned, mocked, jeered, and rejected by those who didn't believe He was who He claimed to be. He also performed many miracles and drew crowds of people who pursued Him only for what they could get from Him. Toward the end of His life and ministry, his closest friends deserted Him. He was also betrayed by one of the disciples in His most intimate circle. Subsequently, He was ruthlessly beaten and scourged by the governing authorities. In the process of fulfilling His earthly mission, "He was despised and rejected by men; a man of sorrows, and acquainted with grief" (Isaiah 53:3). Jesus experienced pain, hunger, fatigue, torture, rejection, frustration, and loneliness so that he could completely identify with the realities of frail humanity. In short, Jesus became like us in every way (see Hebrews 2:17); He did so without sin so that He could be the perfect sacrifice.

Marking his final act of obedience to His Father's will, He was brutally crucified on a cross. (By the way, I wish to point out an often neglected teaching of Scripture: for God to pardon guilty sinners is actually the secondary reason that Jesus died on the cross. As I mentioned earlier, Jesus ultimately went to the cross so that His Father's glory would be put on full display.) In addition to the joy of pleasing His Father, while on the cross, Jesus's focus was steadily fixed on all God's children—His brothers and sisters for all eternity—that would be redeemed through His death (see Hebrews 12:2). One may surmise that God the Father was also consumed by our salvation as He watched His blameless son being crucified; we can never begin to imagine His wrenching agony. I think nothing more powerfully attests to God's faithfulness—that He does what He has said He will do—than this singular event in history. Although He could have, God didn't back down from His original plan of redemption or use His omnipotence to save His beloved Son from suffering a most horrific and despicable death on our behalf.

Jesus "was pierced for our transgressions; he was crushed for our iniquities" (Isaiah 53:5). All of humanity's collective sins—past, present, and future—hammered the nails into His hands and feet; our wretchedness pierced the crown of thorns into His head. As unimaginable and excruciating as this physical pain was, some theologians have speculated that the most agonizing pain Jesus endured was being separated from the eternal fellowship that He had enjoyed with His Father. Yet, willingly and in gross humiliation, Jesus spilled His blood for us, as the Bible teaches that without the shedding of blood there can be no forgiveness of sins (see Leviticus 17:11; Hebrews 9:22). Romans 6:23 states, "For the wages of sin is death but the free gift of God is eternal life through Christ Jesus our Lord." Hence, Jesus's sacrifice forever settled the debt we owed God that we could never, ever pay. Because of the shed blood of Jesus, the Bible declares that though our sins are as scarlet, God has washed us white as snow (see Isaiah 1:18). What unspeakable love! What could endear Christ to us more or make a greater appeal to our gratitude than that which He eternally secured for us by going to the cross? Truly, God demonstrated His extravagant love for us because "He did not spare his own Son but gave him up for us all" (Romans 8:32). "In this is love, not that we have loved God but that he loved us" (1 John 4:10). And "While we were still sinners, Christ died for us" (Romans 5:8). In this one glorious act as the God-man, Jesus once and for all bridged the infinite chasm that had separated man from God due to Adam and Eve's sin.

At the moment of Jesus's final breath, God's eternal purpose to save the lost was accomplished. The veil in the Holy of Holies was torn, signifying that communion between God and man had been decisively restored (see Matthew 27:51). God, the merciful Judge, put down His divine gavel. To those who choose to accept Jesus's sacrifice on their behalf, whose sins have now been forgiven, our verdict reads: no longer guilty—perfectly loved and wholly accepted by the Father. God accomplished this lavish display of grace without ever violating His righteousness or compromising His justice (see 1 Corinthians 1:24). God is infinitely just and gracious because not a single person is deserving of this unspeakably wondrous and beautiful exchange wherein the righteousness of Christ has freely been given to us.

Since enemies don't concern themselves with each other's welfare, it's unthinkable to me that God lovingly sought us out when we were yet His enemies, and that Jesus willingly endured a gruesome death to make a way for the very enemies of God to be reconciled to God (see Romans 5:10; Colossians 1:21). Because the grave could not hold Jesus—because God died in the flesh and literally raised Himself back to life—Jesus's death and glorious resurrection defeated both sin and death. Scripture teaches that Christ now sits at the right hand of His Father in Heaven, interceding for us, and will come back a second time to gather those who are His (see Romans 8:34; Matthew 24:30; Acts 1:11; 1 Corinthians 15:19–23; Revelations 1:7–8). God's Word assures us that one glorious day, our mortal enemy, Satan, will be subdued forever, all things will become subject to the authority of Christ, and He will reign forever as King of Kings and Lord of Lords. Moreover, because of Christ's decisive victory over the grave, those who are His have ultimately conquered death and the tyranny of sin. Our blessed hope is that some great day our mortal bodies will be transformed into immortal bodies, and we will dwell with God forever and ever (see 1 Corinthians 15:51–55; John 14:2–3; Revelations 21:3)!

But it gets even better. Christ has also made those who are His into heirs and joint heirs with Him (see Romans 8:17). Virtually everyone would be flat-out excited were a rich relative to designate him or her as heir to a wealthy estate. If you belong to Christ, you are heir to incredible spiritual blessings and wealth that the world cannot give, and likewise can never take away. How much more elated should we be that Jesus has made us heirs and joint heirs with Him of His everlasting kingdom. The incredible reality of this wondrous inheritance is that God is ours and we are God's forever!

I CHOOSE YOU!

But as great as it is to be heirs of Christ, there's still more: "See how very much our Father loves us, for he calls us his children, and that is what we are!" (1 John 3:1, New Living Translation). This is one of my favorite passages in the Bible because it encapsulates God's extravagant and unfathomable love for us. God "redeem[ed] those who were under the law, so that we might receive adoption as sons" (Galatians 4:5). According to the Bible, this promise is not true of every individual; it is only applicable to those who are the children of God. In light of this glorious truth, a Christian—better yet, follower of Christ—may be defined as a person who knows God as Father. If God is your Father, then you are a treasured son or daughter, indwelled by the spirit of the living God. You should stand in awe and revel that you are a child of the Most High God with all the accompanying rights, privileges, and blessings.

Though it cost God's only Son to willingly be stripped of His glory in order to make us right with God, we have been given something absolutely astonishing—yet it required nothing whatsoever on our part. In giving us this unspeakable gift, God has graciously given us *everything* because He's given us Himself! There was a time when I didn't really understand God's mind-boggling generosity on my behalf. Even though I knew that Christ died for my sins, I didn't truly "get" that the Son of God became incarnate as a man to enable sinful men to become the very children of God. I did not comprehend that I am now doubly God's—not only did He create me but also He has once and for all redeemed me from the dominion of sin and darkness (see

Colossians 1:13); otherwise, I would have experienced everlasting condemnation and eternal separation from His presence. So I think it might be helpful to look more closely at how followers of Christ have come to receive all the temporal, spiritual, and eternal blessings that are now ours to enjoy.

God often uses parallels in life that we can more readily grasp to help us understand deeper spiritual truths. Although these parallels are but a faint echo of the real thing, they can help expand our understanding of spiritual concepts and principles. An example of this is spiritual adoption.

An adoption occurs when a child is handpicked to be the recipient of his adopted family's love. However, we can appreciate the full import of 1 John 3:1, where God calls us his children, only by understanding the concept of adoption during biblical times, which closely paralleled spiritual adoption. In those days, if an adult did not have an heir, he would adopt an adult male son for the sole purpose of carrying on the family name. Imagine a man who had little or nothing one day suddenly inheriting someone else's entire estate. His life would be radically changed.

Although this aspect of adoption is quite foreign to most of us today, we do understand that adopted children are afforded a similar privilege when they are placed into a loving home. Like the adopted male in biblical times, the child also becomes the recipient of a free gift. Therefore, even today's adoption practices can help us appreciate the gravity of what God has done by bringing us into His family.

LIVING AS SONS AND DAUGHTERS

Like adopting males in biblical times and adopting children today, God has adopted those who are His, except His demonstrated kindness is to an infinitely greater degree. Therefore, at the heart of the New Testament message is the incredible truth that we are the adopted children of God. As our adoptive Father, God has plucked us out of the gutter of our sins, rescuing and pardoning us. He has cared for and continues to care for us with a love whose width, length, breadth, and depth we will spend all of eternity trying to fully comprehend (see Ephesians 3:18). That we have a heavenly Father who tenderly cares for us and whose grace, mercy, and compassion cover us is the highest privilege that we could ever have. Also, because He is our Father, we can approach the God of the universe with boldness and confidence as beloved children because the blood of Jesus has made us righteous or blameless in His sight (see Hebrews 10:19–20). This reality is in stark contrast to the sacrificial system of the Old Testament, wherein only the high priest could approach God in the Holy of Holies, and this but once a year (see Hebrews 9:7). Truly, "to be right with God the Judge is a great thing, but to be loved and cared for by God the Father is a greater."[18]

It keeps getting better. As God's children, we have come to share in the very life of Christ. I still can't fathom the idea that God now delights in us and loves us just as He loves Jesus (see John 17:23). But God hasn't adopted us to leave us just the way He found us. No, in adopting us, God desires to transform us as we progressively take on more of His nature and attributes. Hence, the desire of earthly parents to instill positive qualities, values, attitudes, and behaviors in their children—so that they reflect well on the family name—is but a faint whisper of our Father's longing that we increasingly look and act more like Him.

We must grasp once and for all the amazing truth that God freely chose to adopt us into His family. He did so because He simply wanted to, not because it was His duty. Even more incredulous is that, unlike an adoptive parent who might, for example, be smitten by a child's beautiful countenance, we offered God absolutely no compelling reason to adopt us. You see, not only were we completely without merit, we had nothing but our total depravity to offer Him. Nevertheless, God

18. J. I. Packer, *Knowing God* (Downer's Grove: InterVarsity Press, 1973), 207.

reached out in love to forgive us of our sins and to redeem us from the eternal condemnation and wrath that we rightfully deserved. He gave *everything* to make us His sons and daughters.

NO DISNEY STORY CAN TOP THIS

No Disney story, however imaginative or captivating, could ever top what God has done for us. A truth so glorious that John exclaimed, "See how great a love the Father has bestowed on us, that we would be called children of God; and *such* we are" (1 John 3:1, New American Standard Bible). As an adopted child of God, how will I respond to this incomprehensible love that God has lavished on me? How will you respond? I believe that when we truly comprehend what God has done for us, our hearts will be forever changed.

Because our full grasp of our place in God's family is so critical to authentically walking out our faith, it has been aptly said that an accurate knowledge of Christianity is only as sound as one's comprehension of what it means to be adopted into God's family. Hence, the depth and richness of our personal awareness of God as Abba determines to a large extent the zeal that we either manifest or lack as His children. J. I. Packer saliently notes, "If you want to judge how well a person understands Christianity, find out how much he makes of the thought of being God's child, and having God as his Father. If this is not the thought that prompts and controls his worship and prayers and his whole outlook on life, it means that he does not understand Christianity very well at all. For everything that Christ taught, everything that makes the New Testament new, and better than the old, everything that is distinctively Christian as opposed to merely Jewish, is summed up in the knowledge of the Fatherhood of God."[19] (This truth is a good gauge to evaluate our own faith, not a lens to see or critique others' faith.)

---

19. J. I. Packer, *Knowing God* (Downer's Grove: InterVarsity Press, 1973), 201.

Based on my experience, I couldn't agree more. My love and zeal for God deepened only after I had truly apprehended that God was my Father. And this understanding of God as my Father didn't come about until I truly appreciated the lengths that He has gone to in order to make me His child.

GOD'S DESIRED RESPONSE

Until we've grasped the incredible measure of our Father's limitless love for us, we invariably will act like unruly, hardheaded children who are perfectly content to disobey the rules of their father, time and time again. We must take to heart that, as members of God's family and kingdom, submitting to Jesus as our Lord and King is not optional. God's Word instructs: "lead a life worthy of your calling, for you have been called by God" (Ephesians 4:1, New Living Translation). God has set us apart to lead lives worthy of our designation as His sons and daughters. When we fully understand this truth, we will deeply desire to obey our Father and to become more like Him. Both our obedience to Him and our imitation of Him will be reflected in each and every aspect of our lives—our thoughts, conduct, attitude, motives, and behavior.

Because God's unmerited grace has sought us and found us, His desired response is that we would be filled with such adoration and heartfelt gratitude that we can't help but want to passionately love Him in return. He also desires us to be consumed with zeal to live for the praise of His glory. Truth be told, though, we can't display this kind of passion until we have first cultivated a burning love for God. This impassioned love for God seems to be sorely missing in the lives of many disciples today. As a result, many do not—indeed, positively cannot—live in a manner that is glorifying to God.

Before reading further, I hope you will pause and allow God to examine your heart. The reality is that God wants you to experience an ever-deepening love for Him. No matter how ardent our love is now, He wants to empower us to love Him with ever greater abandonment—more devotedly, more single-mindedly, and more unashamedly.

CHAPTER 10

....

BUILDING THE HOUSE OF GOD

You yourselves like living stones are being
built up as a spiritual house.
—1 Peter 2:5

In order to build anything properly—including a significant life—
certain basic steps must be sequentially followed. Indeed, we cannot
ignore the instructions and guidelines set forth if we want to achieve
success. In this chapter, we'll look at the major steps of building a house
to describe how to build a spiritual house that projects God's glory. Just
like a physical structure follows a predetermined blueprint, so must
our spiritual house. That blueprint is Jesus. Scripture admonishes, "For
no one can lay a foundation other than that which is laid, which is
Jesus Christ" (1 Corinthians 3:11). It also teaches that, "the *cornerstone*
is Christ Jesus himself" (Ephesians 2:19–20, New Living Translation;
emphasis mine). Unequivocally, God calls on us to make Christ Jesus
the cornerstone of each and every part of our lives as we purpose to
live backward for the praise of His great name.

EXCAVATION—STUDY OF GOD'S WORD

In the previous chapter, we saw the vital importance of recognizing what God has done in making us His children. This chapter builds on our understanding of God. If we don't care to genuinely know the God who inspired the writing of the Bible, why would we sincerely desire to know or apply what He has revealed in His Word? The fact of the matter is that it's impossible to authentically live for God's honor if we don't study the Bible because Scripture is the primary means whereby the Spirit of God molds and shapes us. It is not enough to simply attend church and only listen to the pastor's sermons—he may lead you astray as he is not free of error or misinterpretation of Scripture. You yourself must be growing in your knowledge of the Bible. Indeed, seeking to know and understand the enduring truths of God's Word should be the hallmark in the life of a true disciple.

Therefore, just as the ground must first be excavated before a house can be built, we must dig into, unearth, and turn over the contents of the Bible. Spiritual excavation involves two steps which absolutely cannot occur absent of the indwelling presence of the Holy Spirit: first, we must understand who God says He is, His nature and attributes; and second, we must understand His Word or counsel as a whole. This enables us to interpret Scripture by Scripture: to understand a passage in light of what the rest of the Scriptures say on that topic. However, unlike the excavation for a physical house—where once completed no further excavation is necessary—we must continue unearthing and mining the treasures in God's Word. Excavation, then, may be likened to the diligent study of the Bible so that we continually grow in our understanding of who God is and what He desires of us.

Written more than three thousand years ago by the inspiration of the Holy Spirit, the Bible is God's infallible revelation of Himself. God invites us to study the Bible because without a clear and accurate understanding of His true character, our spiritual house is bound to eventually sway and buckle under the weight of human errors, presumptions, and misconceptions not only about God but also about ourselves and the world in which we live. Similarly, if we don't understand scriptural precepts and principles, we simply cannot know how God desires us to live. God's Word is the only absolute and authoritative standard for truth. I've heard it said that the BIBLE is our Basic Instructions Before Leaving Earth; it is our Creator's user manual for us—we were *never* designed to go through life without reliance on Him. Therefore, we must heed His counsel. It's important to point out that failure to study the Bible is one of the biggest reasons that we lose our way; for the most part, it is choosing to ignore guidance from the divine GPS. Being off course opens us to greater temptations and assaults from the enemy, undermines our true purpose, and short-circuits God's power in our lives. All in all, an inaccurate understanding of both God and His Word directly affects the degree to which Christ is exalted in our lives.

As we delve into the Word, the Spirit of God brings about a pivotal shift that awakens our desire to love God; eventually, God changes our weak yearning to know and pursue Him to a more vigorous one. Also, as we study God's Word and allow it to take root in our hearts, the work of the Holy Spirit can more easily excavate the things hidden in the recesses of our hearts that have no place in Gods' kingdom. He uncovers and removes them as we yield ourselves to the piercing light of Truth and steadfastly resolve to follow God's will. Besides studying Scripture, we must also seek the Holy Spirit's help to continually move nuggets of the soil of biblical knowledge from our heads and deposit them in our hearts.

Those nuggets must be firmly planted in order to uproot false beliefs and misperceptions—this can't be overemphasized. To give mere mental assent to Scripture is not the same as applying it to our lives. Any biblical knowledge that we attain is of no true benefit if it isn't applied. This is why James 1:22 teaches, "But be doers of the word, and not hearers only, deceiving yourselves." God's Word becomes a part of us only as we purpose to put it into practice. Indeed, knowledge must journey from our heads to our hearts before it can begin to influence our thoughts and, subsequently, our actions. Otherwise, we simply will not be empowered to change what we think and what we do.

For example, in seeking to be more like Christ Jesus, there's often a gap between what we know in our head about who Christ is and our actual conduct. We must go beyond giving only mental assent to the truth that "if anyone is in Christ, he is a new creation. The old has passed away; behold, the new has come" (2 Corinthians 5:17). It must go from our heads to our hearts that we literally possess the very life of Christ; that the same resurrection power that raised Jesus Christ from the grave indwells us, empowering us to fulfill God's will for our lives. Then by faith and with the help of the Holy Spirit, we must take what we intellectually know of Christ—for example, that He is loving and merciful—and then translate those attributes into our actual experience so that in practice, we progressively become more loving and more merciful. However, this is not to say that we fake our way, for example, into merely acting loving. Rather, we are called to *be* loving because Christ in us *is* loving. This typically gradual process is essentially how people with sinful desires and selfish interests come to progressively reflect the nature of God.

Because this process of head-to-heart understanding is of paramount importance in our lives, God also gives us a rich promise as we study His Word: "but the one who looks into the perfect law, the law of liberty, and perseveres, *being no hearer who forgets but a doer who acts*, he will be blessed in his doing" (James 1:25; emphasis mine). God underscores this promise: "He rewards those who seek him" (Hebrews 11:6).

Contrary to what many tend to believe, scriptural commands are not burdensome. Instead, they can be likened to guardrails that help keep us on God's path for our lives, much like physical guardrails keep us from careening out of control or driving off a cliff. As we gain an accurate understanding of God's commands and apply them to our lives, we grow spiritually. And as we come to know how God sees us, we also grow in our love for Him, causing our desires to change so that following His commands and fleeing from sin increasingly becomes a delight. Through this process, we learn how to progressively honor our Creator and experience His best for our lives. It cannot be overstated that the study of God's Word is at the heart of cultivating a passion for His glory.

The amazing reality is that God has graciously promised to bless and reward us for spending time with Him in His Word. Many of these wonderful blessings and rewards will be ours to enjoy in this temporal life. While many of them will not be experienced here on earth, by making the most of the gift of hindsight and living backward, they, nonetheless, will be ours to delight in for all eternity.

LAYING A FIRM FOUNDATION — CULTIVATING HUMILITY

After the excavation has been completed, the foundation of the house is then laid. In many respects, the foundation is the most important element of a structure. Because everything else rests on it, getting the foundation right is critical. Just like the foundation of a physical house ultimately determines how stable the house will be, understanding ourselves in relation to God is fundamental to the structural integrity of our spiritual house. This spiritual attribute is called humility, and it facilitates the essential heart change that enables us to acknowledge our need of God.

As the penetrating light of God's truth opens the eyes of our hearts, we are enabled to better understand His glorious attributes. At the same time, God exposes our true nature. We then discover our deep-rooted pride and self-confidence. We become more aware of our imperfections—frailties, weaknesses, and shortcomings. We also see the remnants of corruption still lurking in our hearts. This exposure of who we really are enables us to grasp why we need God's Word, while also showing us our desperate need for His transforming grace and mercy. As a result of this illuminating process, our self-confidence and inflated view of ourselves begin to progressively shrink. Conversely, we see God in His greatness, and grasp that as the Lord over the entire universe, He is sovereignly directing and controlling all things for His purposes and for the display of His glory—and lo, we are not. Our recognition of this truth humbles us, proverbially cutting us down to size. The result is that we apprehend our proper position in relation to God: He is the Creator and we are His creatures; He is everything to us and, without Him, we are less than nothing.

But it's critical that we have a balanced view of humility. It is false humility to continually focus on the fact that we are nothing without God—because the glorious truth is that, in Christ Jesus, God now sees us as holy, perfect, and blameless. "For our sake he [God] made him [Jesus] to be sin who knew no sin, so that in him we might become the righteousness of God" (2 Corinthians 5:21). Yet at the same time to not acknowledge and be ever mindful that we are nothing without God— that it's only by His grace that we are what we are—leads to pride and thinking way too highly of ourselves. Scripture gives this warning, "Don't think you are better than you really are" (Romans 12:3, New Living Translation). In other words, don't be prideful. Examples of pride are when we are more concerned about gaining man's approval than doing what we know God would have us do, when we see ourselves as better or holier than others, and when we take personal credit for the abilities, strengths, and accomplishments God has given to us. Although in and of ourselves we have absolutely nothing to offer God—because even our best acts of righteousness or goodness are as filthy rags in His sight (see Isaiah 64:6)—God sees us as worthy. Not because of who we are in and of ourselves, but only because He has chosen to make us His treasures.

However, this is not to say that there isn't a "right" or healthy way to love ourselves for who we are. After all, God Himself loves us despite all our sins and baggage. What I mean is that our confidence or sense of importance must always be rooted in *who* we are (forgiven and free) and *whose* we are (God's) because of the finished work of Christ's sacrifice. This awareness of God's perfect acceptance of us enables us to freely embrace 1 John 1:9: "If we confess our sins, he is faithful and just to forgive us our sins and to cleanse us from all unrighteousness." Some abuse the grace of God and use this Scripture to wantonly indulge their sinful desires. However, this teaching absolutely does not give license to sin (see Romans 6:1–4); neither does it mean that we should not be contrite for our transgressions against God. Indeed, there's a right or biblical place for brokenness and heartfelt remorse for our sins (see Psalm 51:17).

Yet I know from experience that there's a natural tendency to inordinately dwell on our failures and shortcomings and to feel condemned, even after we've confessed our sins and have been forgiven by God. This proclivity certainly delights the enemy of our souls as it is opposed to the grace and freedom that God desires us to live in. So there needs to be a healthy tension between being sorry for our sins and boldly walking in freedom. In other words, instead of being overly preoccupied about what we've done wrong (or are still getting wrong), God's unconditional acceptance empowers us to move past confessed sins and to focus primarily on our spiritual growth—on the good things that He is accomplishing in and through us.

However, even after we've seen ourselves in proper relation to God, pride and self-sufficiency persist in our hearts. As we cultivate humility, though, we progressively grow in our dependence on God and look to Him for everything as we increasingly put less stock in our own goodness, self-efforts, and abilities. This dynamic is the essence of humility; it's why humility is the foundation of our spiritual house. Just as there can be no stable house without a foundation, there can be no spiritual growth without humility; without humility, we'll continue to be blinded to the true spiritual condition of our hearts or just how messed up we really are absent of God's inner workings in us. Though saved by *redeeming* grace, we often lack motivation to pursue the godly attributes God desires for our lives simply because we don't see the necessity for godly change in our lives. We don't see our continued desperate need for God's *transforming* grace, which empowers us to align our lives with His will.

Therefore, a heart posture of humility is the means by which all other spiritual virtues are birthed and cultivated (see 1 Peter 1:16). The crux of the matter is this: where there is little or no humility, there is little or no suppleness of heart. Where there is little or no suppleness of heart, there is little or no molding of our hearts. Where there is little or no molding, God receives little or no glory from our lives. So for our continued growth in Christ, humility is our closest ally, and pride is our worst enemy. As such, humility is indeed the foundation upon which our lives are built up in Christ and thus securely established.

FRAMING AND ROOFING THE HOUSE — CULTIVATING THE FEAR OF GOD

Framing a house is the process of creating the frame or skeleton on which the other parts of the house will be hung. It must be structurally sound, as it gives shape and support to the house. We frame our spiritual house with a genuine, reverential fear of God because it shapes and supports our understanding of our Father's heart and His purpose for our lives. But there can be no understanding of God without a sound fear of God. Scripture teaches, "The fear of the Lord is the *beginning of knowledge*; fools despise wisdom and instruction" (Proverbs 1:7, emphasis mine). Knowledge, in this verse, refers to knowing God. Therefore, without a reverential fear of God, it's simply impossible to genuinely know God and, in turn, walk out His will for our lives.

What exactly does it mean to fear God? When the Bible mentions the fear of God, it is referring to a profound sense of awe and veneration toward Him. I like how Jerry Bridges puts it: "There is an infinite gap in worth and dignity between God the Creator and man the creature, even though man has been created in the image of God. The fear of God is a heartfelt recognition of this gap—not a putdown of man, but an exaltation of God."[20]

According to a multitude of Scriptures, this deep respect and reverence for God should pervade our entire outlook on life, as Jesus modeled for us when He was on the earth (see Isaiah 11:1–3; Acts 9:31; Colossians 3:22; 2 Corinthians 7:1; 1 Peter 2:17). It should condition our motives, motivate us to make God-honoring choices and decisions, and influence all that we think, say, and do. However, I would not be providing an accurate description of the fear of God if I neglected to mention that, because we still fall short of Gods glory, we should also harbor a holy awareness of His temporal judgments against sin. Even though those who belong to Christ have ultimately been delivered from the wrath of God, we are still at His mercy for the potential immediate consequences of our sin as well as His fatherly discipline. Thus, reverential fear is a catalyst for becoming contrite and repentant for the sins we commit against a holy God. It also helps us to be broken of our self-will as we purpose to surrender our desires to Christ. I know from experience that this brokenness always precedes our desire to passionately pursue God, and indeed we can never be broken before Him, let alone begin to honor Him, without this reverential fear.

Moreover, if we do not have a healthy fear of God, we will naturally gravitate toward one of two negative extremes: a servile apprehension of God—exhibiting the kind of anxious dread that a child has of a harshly demanding parent who is difficult to please; or a very casual relationship with God—displaying the sort of absent fear that a child has toward a parent who is overly lenient and rarely or never administers discipline. In the first scenario, we would view God as overly demanding or as someone whom we can never satisfy; we'll also see Him as eagerly wanting to punish us for our smallest inability to abide by His many "impossible" rules and demands. In the latter case, our view is just the opposite. Having little or no anticipation of God's

20. Jerry Bridges, *The Practice of Godliness* (Colorado Springs: NavPress, 2008), 23.

displeasure, we will tend to be flippant and presumptuous in our relationship with Him. As the daughter I'm blessed with wisely observed, the second scenario is as if this parent would say, "If you don't stop— I'm going to do nothing." Thus, a healthy tension must exist between our reverential fear of God and our childlike confidence in Him as a good and loving Father. And since we've seen that God does all things to uphold His great glory, we exhibit a healthy fear of God when we see His goodness as being secondary to His greatness.

When our knowledge of God is rooted in reverential fear, then the proper end of all understanding is that we may know God and stand in awe of Him. Any other pursuit of knowledge, biblical or otherwise, is ultimately meaningless. Jesus affirmed this when He declared, "And this is *eternal life, that they know you the only true God, and Jesus Christ* whom you have sent" (John 17:3; emphasis mine).

Reverential fear enables us to get a closer look at the God of the universe. It gives us a magnified view of God that enables us to better understand His glorious attributes—His vastness, greatness, majesty, omnipotence, splendor, omniscience, unparalleled beauty, infinite goodness, magnificent love, omnipresence, unfathomable mercy, immeasurable love, unending compassion, holy justice, and righteous wrath. A deeper understanding of all God's attributes helps us to magnify and exalt Him with increasing vigor. On the contrary, to perceive or relate to God through the lens of our restricted comprehension amounts to thinking miniscule thoughts of an infinitely immense and awesome God who has declared, "For my thoughts are not your thoughts, neither are your ways my ways" (Isaiah 55:8). Therefore, reverential fear also reins in our natural affinity for making erroneous assumptions about God based on our limited understanding. As such, it is the only antidote for thinking small thoughts of God.

In addition, the degree to which we display an awe of God is the only accurate index of how God-centered our views truly are. Thus, we can know that we're actually growing in our fear of God as we increasingly resist our natural tendency to have a man-centered outlook on life. I encourage you to make the practical outworking of this truth your yardstick as you seek to grow in the fear of God. Jesus taught, "For to everyone who has will more be given, and he will have an abundance. But from the one who has not, even what he has will be taken away" (Matthew 25:29; see also Luke 19:14–26). This principle applies to reverential fear. As we learn to fear and esteem God, the deeper and richer our knowledge of him becomes; the deeper and richer our knowledge, the more deeply we fear and esteem Him. This dynamic leads to greater intimacy; it also promotes our devotion to God. Conversely, if we are remiss in delving into understanding God through His Word, we'll know less of His awesome attributes, not understand His true heart for us, and forfeit intimacy. All of these result in a loss of the Lord's presence and power in our lives.

I've also discovered that our awe of God circuitously increases our love for Him and fosters a zeal to live set apart for His glory. Therefore, although many of us have not made this connection, learning to approach God with an attitude of awe and reverence is foundational to finding true significance in life; it's a critical component of living backward. Without it, we will encounter major roadblocks in pleasing God. After all, only a person with a healthy reverential fear of God can fully apprehend His lavish grace toward us and thus desire to please Him by living a life of holiness. As John Murray noted, "The fear of God is the soul of godliness."[21]

So before moving on to the next step in this spiritual building process, let's briefly discuss how to cultivate a reverential fear of God. Proverbs 2:1–6 provides a concise answer. It instructs us to *accept* God's words and *store up* His commands within us by *turning* our ears to wisdom and *applying* our hearts to understanding. It also teaches that if we *cry out* for insight and understanding and *search* for it as hidden treasure, then we will *understand* the fear of the Lord and *find* knowledge of God. For the Lord gives wisdom, and from His mouth

---

21. Cited in Jerry Bridges, *The Practice of Godliness* (Colorado Springs: NavPress, 2008), 25.

comes knowledge and understanding. Each of the italicized verbs above refers to humbly coming into alignment with God's will. It's by heeding these admonitions that we come to fear the Lord and gain knowledge of Him. Inherent in these instructions is also a promise that *if* we diligently pursue wisdom, we *will* understand the fear of God; we will come to intimately know God.

FEAR OF GOD CARRIES OTHER PROMISES

But there are other intangible benefits of fearing God. You may recall me mentioning earlier that I find joy and delight living in God's presence. Well, reverential fear birthed this desire and continues to nurture it. Strange as it might seem, joy is a wonderful by-product of fearing God. Moreover, many passages of Scripture teach that God delights in favoring and blessing those who exhibit reverential fear toward Him. Psalm 31:19 is but one of such verses that attests to this: "How great is your goodness, which you have stored up for those who fear you." (See also Psalms 34:9–10, 103:13, 112:1, 115:13, 128:1–4 for more examples.)

Let's quickly look at two of these blessings.

ON THE DIVINE JUMBOTRON

In one of my favorite Scriptures, God declares, "Heaven is my throne, and the earth is my footstool . . . All these things my hand has made, and so all these things came to be, declares the Lord. But this is the one to whom I will look: *he who is humble and contrite in spirit and trembles at my word*" (Isaiah 66:1–2; emphasis mine). According to this Scripture, there's something we can do—or a way we can be—that attracts the attention of the God of the universe. The "magnet" that captures God's attention, drawing His gaze toward us, is a heart adorned with humility—a heart bowed in recognition of its desperate need for Him and that beats with reverential awe. Referring back to the Jumbotron example mentioned in the beginning of this book, walking in the fear of God is like being on the divine Jumbotron of the audience of one! I don't know about you, but this is the screen that I want to always appear on; really, it's the only one worth truly getting excited about.

FRIENDS OF GOD

I think every sincere follower of Christ desires to be a friend of God, yet I also believe that many of us don't understand what this friendship means. Who exactly is a friend of God? We can answer this question by looking at Abraham, whom God referred to as His friend (see James 2:23). Abraham was accorded this commendation because he obeyed God, as demonstrated by his willingness to risk his security, comfort, reputation, and future based on what God had commanded him: namely, to leave his homeland and go to an unspecified place (see Genesis 12:1–20). Abraham also received this honor because he had a rock-solid trust in God. When God required him to choose between his love for God and his love for his beloved son, Isaac—the son God had given him despite being in old age and past the ability to father a child—Abraham chose God. In humility and obedience to God, he was literally willing to sacrifice Isaac (see Genesis 22). This act of obedience is even more remarkable given that Isaac was the son through whom God had promised Abraham that his descendants would outnumber the grains of sand on the seashore. Abraham believed that, no matter what, God somehow would remain true to His promise.

Through both of these actions, Abraham demonstrated that he was a true worshiper of God. Essentially, it was his reverential fear of God that enabled him to both trust and obey God, ultimately qualifying him as a friend of God. The God of the universe is still looking for true worshipers—those with hearts abandoned like Abraham, not only willing to risk all to obey and trust Him but also ready to surrender to Him that which they most love and cherish. For those who do, the blessings in store are beyond their wildest imagination.

Lastly, just as a roof provides protection from physical elements such as wind and rain, a reverential fear of God provides covering and protection against negative spiritual elements that undermine a God-centered outlook. These include such things as storms precipitated by self-centered absorption, rains of thinking far too highly of ourselves, winds of self-confidence, squalls of self-sufficiency, tornadoes of worldly values and false ideas, and the hurricanes of thinking much too small thoughts of God.

ROUGHING IN THE HOUSE—
INFUSING WISDOM INTO OUR LIVES

We've so far covered a two-step excavation process of knowing God and His Word, laying a solid foundation with humility, and framing/roofing our spiritual house with reverential fear. This brings us to the next step of roughing in the house, which refers to the initial installation of all the wiring elements needed to circulate power throughout the house. We rough in our spiritual house with wisdom. As with obtaining knowledge, the fear of God also facilitates the attaining of wisdom (see Proverbs 1:7). Distinct from a vital knowledge of God, wisdom connotes the ability to apply biblical knowledge to our life circumstances so as to achieve the most God-exalting results. Therefore, knowledge and wisdom must work in tandem if we are to truly honor God with our lives. The fact that an entire chapter in the Bible (Proverbs) is dedicated solely to wisdom principles underscores its importance. Just as a house not properly roughed in lacks the "essentials" of heat and electricity, a spiritual house without wisdom lacks the power or know-how for victorious living.

Scripture clearly teaches that if we want to experience God's best—and live a meaningful, victorious, and enduring life of significance—wisdom is the principal thing. According to Proverbs 4:7–8 (New Living Translation), "Getting wisdom is the wisest thing you can do! And whatever else you do, develop good judgment. If you prize wisdom, she will make you great. Embrace her, and she will honor you." (See also Proverbs 3:13–18.) Proverbs 3:15 says of wisdom, "She is more precious than jewels, and nothing you desire can compare with her." Truth be told, though, many of us are far more desirous of temporary precious jewels than we are of enduring wisdom. But if God places such a high value on the importance of obtaining wisdom, then so should we. Proverbs 4:11 shows us that wisdom is our guide: "I have taught you the way of wisdom; I have led you in the paths of uprightness." A similar teaching instructs, "I am the Lord your God, who teaches you what is good for you, and leads you along the paths you should follow" (Isaiah 48:17, New Living Translation). Clearly, we must make a choice as to the paths we will pursue in this temporal life.

Ultimately, there are only two paths. One is God's path—the wise or "straight" path. Guided by the divine GPS, we experience God's promise of blessings, protection, and favor as we walk in His commands (see Isaiah 41:10; Psalms 23:1–4, 48:14, 121:7–8; 2 Corinthians 2:14). The other is man's path—the foolish or crooked path, which often leads in the opposite direction of where God desires us to go (see Psalm 1:1–6). Without a doubt, to varying degrees this crooked path causes us to get turned around and to lose our way. Which of us doesn't desire the rich benefits of walking on the path that is blessed by God? Which of us would purposefully reject the contentment and joy that this path offers? Yet many Christians unwittingly forfeit this blessed contentment, day after day, month after month, year after year.

Ask yourself, "Which path am I pursuing?" If it's not God's path, think about how many of God's rich blessings you've relinquished by going your own way. Although God desires to bless us for walking the straight path, we must understand that He desires us to pursue wisdom first and foremost so that He may be glorified in our lives. This is another clear example of God's glory and our welfare being intertwined. For certain, those who purposefully seek wisdom as life's greatest treasure are the ones who live a truly blessed and meaningful life. Again, we should be most thankful that, as God would mercifully have it, anything that displays His glory in our lives is at the same time intended to bring about our greatest possible good.

THE OUTWORKING OF WISDOM AND REVERENTIAL FEAR

Practically speaking, what does the pursuit of wisdom and reverential fear look like in our lives? Essentially, a healthy fear of God has helped me to become increasingly aware that at all times and in all places, He is ever worthy of my most honorable conduct. Taking this to heart over time has exerted a continual influence on my speech, my attitude, and my behavior, making them progressively more pleasing to God. In a similar vein, besides helping me to make godly choices, wisdom teachings have helped shape each and every aspect of my life. For example, it influences my interactions with others. Having internalized that a soft answer turns away wrath (see Proverbs 15:1) has helped me to remain calm under pressure on countless occasions, diffusing situations that had all the makings to potentially become very heated and unpleasant.

I believe that another most critical outworking of reverential fear is seeking to walk in integrity before God. For example, when recently complimented for something I hadn't done, I spoke up and told my peers that I didn't deserve to receive credit, as I hadn't been responsible. Even though they would have never known I wasn't deserving of the commendation, God *knew*. This death to self (by not courting man's praise) was the result of years having taken to heart a truth that we all tend to so easily overlook: God is most concerned not about what we "do" for Him, but about who we are becoming in Christ. However, I remember when that wasn't the case in my life. In fact, I recall times when my motive for doing certain things wasn't even about honoring God—it was more about gaining man's approval.

Scripture explicitly teaches us to not be concerned with man's superficial opinion of us, but rather, our conduct in the eyes of a holy God. No doubt, this entails obedience to what we know God desires of us, regardless of the response—acceptance or rejection, honor or dishonor, praise or blame—that our words or actions might engender from man. Moreover, John 12:42 instructs us to not love praise from man more than praise from God. I've now learned that decisions become a whole lot easier when our will to please God outweighs our desire to please others.

Scripture also says, "For it is not the one who commends himself who is approved, but the one whom the Lord commends" (2 Corinthians 10:18; see also Galatians 1:10). We must embrace that any commendation conferred by man is worthless if it is not accompanied by the commendation of Almighty God. As followers of Christ, we must pray to come to a place in our spiritual walk where we emphatically declare, as did Peter and the other apostles, "We must obey God rather than men" (Acts 5:29). John Bunyan captured this idea: "If my life is fruitless, it doesn't matter who praises me, and if my life is fruitful, it doesn't matter who criticizes me." Although difficult, it is very freeing when we learn to cast aside what others think of us so long as our God is pleased. To live any differently is to have a greater fear of man the created than God the Creator.

As we seek to walk in integrity, it helps to remember that our reputation is only based on who people think we are, hence the saying, "Integrity is who you are when no one is watching." Our character is who we really are and only God accurately knows that. Whereas to others our reputation is a mere dot-to-dot outline, to God our character is a full-color illustration with an infinite number of megapixels. A reputation based solely on worldly standards may be as brass, but godly character is truly more priceless than gold. Along these lines, honesty in our business dealings and in all that we say and do is an offshoot of upright character (see Proverbs 11:1, 20:23).

Besides seeking to walk in integrity and growing in godly character, a short list of what the pursuit of wisdom and fearing God have practically wrought in my life includes: possessing a strong desire to keep a pure heart before God (see Psalm 24:4), for example, not harboring an offense against someone because even though they aren't aware of it, God is and this attitude negatively affects my fellowship with Him; becoming more transparent, which has resulted in a willingness to confess my sins to others (see James 5:16), for example, becoming more and more comfortable sharing less than glamorous personal information about myself; purposing to do all things without murmuring or complaining (see Philippians 2:14) and not complaining even quietly to myself because, though no one else can hear me, God can; being more determined to not be critical or judgmental of others but to look for the good in them instead (see Luke 6:37); resolving to do all things with excellence as unto the Lord (see Colossians 3:23), whether or not I anticipate receiving man's credit; being continuously challenged to neither exaggerate nor minimize the truth in my conversations with others (see Ephesians 4:15, 25), as this leads to hypocrisy; and being empowered to not take matters into my own hands by either being resentful or acting spitefully when others have mistreated me (see Romans 12:19), as when I want to hold back my love from someone because they have hurt me. Truly, a reverence for God influences each and every aspect of our growth in godliness. And this truth leads us to the next step.

INSULATION AND DRYWALL—THE PURSUIT OF HOLINESS

The next step in the building process is insulation, which protects the house from cold temperatures, followed by installation of the drywall, used to construct the walls and ceilings. This interior work of our spiritual house is analogous to working holiness into each and every aspect of our lives. Not only does holiness insulate us from the onslaught of the world and from our love for God growing cold, but, like walls compartmentalize a house, it should hang from every nook and cranny of our hearts. God has given us His indwelling presence so that we may walk in holiness before Him, not to enlarge our sense of pride and self-sufficiency. If that were the case, we might be tempted to give credit to ourselves for our ability to overcome sin.

In fact, the primary reason that we fail to appropriate more of God's effectual power in our day-to-day struggles with sin and temptations is precisely because of this ingrained sense of self-sufficiency. We instinctively think we can handle life and the situations we face on our own, so we don't look to God for help. This attitude is like missing a turn; left uncorrected due to rebellion or stubbornness, it hinders and sometimes even prevents us from fulfilling God's unique plan for our lives. God desires us to overcome sin by depending more and more on His strength and less and less on our own. This is why He dismantles our perceived self-sufficiency and brings us to the end of ourselves— He allows us to experience failure in order to recognize our need of Him. When we choose to depend on the Holy Spirit's power within us to overcome temptations and sins, He empowers us to experience victory. These triumphs are a source of joy. While there's nothing wrong with feeling good about our ability to conquer sin in dependence on the Lord, this sense of satisfaction should be an outgrowth of our sincere desire to please God rather than the by-product of our pride and self-sufficiency. It should always be an expression of our obedience to God and our awareness of His work in our lives.

EXTERIOR TOUCHES—THE DISPLAY OF HIS GLORY

The next major step is the house's exterior. Its look and finish says volumes about the house and, for good or bad, reflects on the builder.

Similarly, our lives are intended to showcase our Creator. God desires to be involved with every aspect of our spiritual house so that our lives may reflect His glory. He has not infused us with His power and strength as well as promised us His effectual help for any more fundamental reason than this. Ultimately, we have God's indwelling Spirit animating us for *His* power to be known and shown, not ours! Our lives should be all about putting Christ on display.

INTERIOR FINISHING TOUCHES — DECORATING WITH THE FRUIT OF THE SPIRIT

The final major step is outfitting the house's interior. Besides making the house livable, interior furnishings enhance its overall beauty. Wood floors, cabinetry, and appliances add appeal and pizzazz. Lights and area rugs accentuate and highlight focal points. Similarly, as we bring forth more fruit of the Spirit, our spiritual dwelling place increasingly becomes more beautiful and pleasing to God. As a result, we radiate the light of Christ all the more. We become more and more beautiful from the inside out. People see a difference in how we engage life. They notice that our demeanor and conduct are distinctly different and sense the warmth that our countenance exudes. Though they may not know what to attribute it to, they also see the fruit of the Spirit that we manifest—they see that we are more loving, less impatient, more humble, less critical, less self-absorbed, and have genuine joy and peace. As we humbly take less and less of God's blessings for granted, people take notice of our gratitude and praise to God. They are ever watching us, taking note of our faith and trust in God (or lack thereof) when we face trials and difficulties, often calling us out when we come across as imposters. In short, we walk out our calling as true ambassadors of Christ as we make His name great—the world sees our good works and glorifies our Father in Heaven (see Matthew 5:16).

Yet we must always bear in mind that anything good that ever comes *out* of us is only because of Jesus *in* us. And our hearts must remain continually grateful for all God's blessings and for all that He empowers us to do.

Practicing gratitude is a key way to fortify our spiritual house. That is the subject of the next chapter.

CHAPTER 11

....

GRATITUDE FUELS OUR JOY

*Gratitude is lifting a cup filled to the brim with
heartfelt praise and thanksgiving to God . . . and in
the lifting, joy is spilled all over the heart. Gratitude is
the heart posture that fills our lives with joy.*

Gratitude gives us access to joy, and the more gratitude we have, the
deeper our joy will be. This reality is rooted in Scripture—God has
revealed to us how to experience His abiding joy. In this chapter, we'll
delve into the nuts and bolts of how to cultivate more gratitude in
our lives because gratitude not only enlarges our passion for God, it
also results in a joyful heart that decisively points to God and thus
magnifies His glory.

Although it may not always appear this way to our human understanding, day after day God continues to give us no less than His very
best. I've discovered that even in those times when God said no to
what I petitioned Him for, those nos were in reality sacred moments
of grace—they were some of God's greatest acts of love and mercy
toward me. For example, there was a time when I had hoped (maybe
even prayed) for a specific luxury vehicle. I later realized that had
God granted this desire, it may have been the start of wanting other

trappings of success. This preoccupation would have then pulled my focus away from Him. My loving Father denied me what I had thought I needed, as it would have undermined both my continued spiritual growth and my complete devotion to Him. I now embrace the fact that God is good both when He withholds and when He gives. Yet, to my dismay, I find that even when the evidence of God's tender mercies and good gifts are right before my very eyes—like when He gets me safely from point A to point B, when I'm surprised by unexpected good news, when I complete a grueling physical workout, or when I recover from an upper respiratory infection—I at times still fail to acknowledge and thank Him for His goodness. Other times I do only in retrospect.

Maybe it's because I don't see God in physical form as I do humans, whom I'm sure to thank for anything done on my behalf. It disturbs me greatly that I am not as deeply thankful as I want to be to the God who blesses and sustains me in ways that I can never possibly know. I know I'm not alone. Nevertheless, just because we're prone to be unthankful does not absolve us of expressing gratitude to God. In fact, throughout Scripture, God explicitly commands us to offer him both our praise and thanks (see 1 Chronicles 16:34; Psalms 95:2–3, 100:4). With the Lord's help, those occasions when I'm aware of His goodness but not always careful to give Him thanks and praise have become fewer and fewer. The by-product of this grateful attitude is that I'm progressively experiencing more of His joy. And so can you.

In learning how to cultivate a spirit of gratitude, we'll first look at why God commands us to give thanks. Then we'll explore four often overlooked reciprocal spiritual dynamics that sequentially lead us to experiencing more joy.

WE DESERVE NOTHING

Before addressing why God commands us to be thankful, we must lay the groundwork. Remember, in and of ourselves, we are wholly unworthy and absolutely undeserving of anything good from God. Anything God has given us comes from the kind hands of His grace. What's more, because we deserve absolutely nothing from God, nothing that He graciously gives us should ever be regarded as a small blessing. Without a grasp of these two truths, we will neither acknowledge God's countless gifts nor give thanks to Him for them. On the contrary, an understanding of these truths enables us to appreciate why God commands us to give Him our heartfelt thanks.

Psalm 106:1 declares, "Praise the Lord. Oh give thanks to the Lord, for he is good, for his steadfast love endures forever!" In fact in Psalm 136 alone, the command to give thanks to God occurs twenty-six times! Throughout Scripture, we see that God desires His people to declare their gratitude to Him for His goodness and loving kindness. Why does He? Besides the fact that He is immeasurably worthy of our praise and thanks, the most fundamental reason God calls us to give Him thanks is that it is part of our act of worship. Thus, it is integral to glorifying Him with our lives (see Romans 12:1). As we offer thanks to God for His good gifts, we are better able to recognize His fatherly care in our lives, which then draws us nearer to His heart. Truly, there's no better place than to be near to God's heart, experiencing deep intimacy with the Lover of our souls!

There was a time when I thought that expressing my thanks to God was something I had to always speak aloud. While I'm not in any way minimizing the fact that we are called to express gratitude to God with the fruit of our lips (see Psalm 28:7; Hebrews 13:15), I now know that because God knows our thoughts before we even speak them (see Psalm 139:4), even a silent thought of gratitude touches His heart. The same holds true for worship and praise.

I mentioned earlier that I'm fond of saying, "God is the 'goodest,'" to underscore just how good He is. As we recognize just how completely undeserving we are of any of God's good gifts, we begin to more deeply appreciate our utter dependence on Him for everything in life. This brings us to the first of four spiritual dynamics that enable us to experience more of God's joy, namely, *a greater understanding of our utter unworthiness leads to a greater dependence on God.*

Experience has taught me that the degree to which we recognize our dependence on God and see all blessings as graciously coming from Him is an accurate index of our humility.

Have you ever by accident tried to capture an image by looking through the wrong end of a camera's viewfinder? I have. It's simply not possible. This illustrates the inability of the proud and arrogant—who lack humility—to see or understand their own depravity. They simply cannot recognize their very desperate need of God. Conversely, and as discussed in the previous chapter, the humble keenly grasp their great need of God; they are deeply aware of their dependence on Him for all that they are and all that they have. This awareness fosters an even greater humility toward God, as seen in the next spiritual dynamic: *a greater dependence on God leads to greater humility and less arrogance.*

PRIDE SMOTHERS GRATITUDE

Besides arrogant people's inability to recognize their need of God, they typically are ungrateful. Henry Ward Beecher said, "Pride slays thanksgiving . . . a proud man is seldom a grateful man, for he never thinks he gets as much as he deserves." So true! In general, arrogant people are ungrateful for the simple reason that neither can they see God's goodness nor realize just how undeserving they are of His gifts. They do not grasp just how very different their lives would be without God's grace and countless blessings. In contrast, the attitude of a thankful heart is generally borne out of the recognition that God gives it what it does not deserve. Grateful people recognize that God chooses to bless them not because He needs to but because He graciously desires to. In fact, if God were to do nothing else for us (though the very idea itself contradicts God's giving nature), we would still be immeasurably indebted to Him. So when we mistakenly feel entitled to God's blessings, we greatly diminish His goodness. This attitude dishonors God—when we act as though God is obligated to bless us, we exalt our deservedness over His goodness. On the contrary, practicing gratitude fosters a deepening humility and helps to counteract the sin of pride.

CONDUCTORS OF GRACE

This brings us to our third reciprocal spiritual dynamic. Just like arrogance spawns ingratitude, there's a direct relationship between gratitude and humility: the more thankful a person is toward God, the more humble he/she will be. Therefore, grateful people are generally humble people. The more the humble grasp how greatly they are at the mercy of God, the more clearly they see His goodness in their lives, recognize His unmerited blessings, and offer Him heartfelt thanks. Indeed, it is in the soil of humility that the virtue of thankfulness grows and thrives.

The opposite scenario is true. Without humility, the thankfulness of our hearts toward God is prone to wither. This is because the essence of pride is to think and act independently of God. After all, why is it necessary to acknowledge or thank God when one mistakenly believes that any success or good thing in life is the result of his/her own efforts and abilities? So just like independence from God is an index of arrogance, the extent to which we fail to thank God for His good gifts generally reveals the extent of our pride. The relationship between gratitude and humility is seen in this dynamic: *greater humility fosters increased gratitude and vice versa.*

It is to our great detriment to downplay the reality that where there is little or no gratitude toward God, there is also little or no humility. Scripture emphatically teaches, "God opposes the proud, but gives grace to the humble" (James 4:6; 1 Peter 5:5). It also issues this solemn warning, "Pride goes before destruction, and a haughty spirit before a fall" (Proverbs 16:18). Too often, we give these Scriptures only mental assent. Yet we've seen that pride is a snare and extremely dangerous to our spiritual well-being. When we act in ways that are prideful, we foolhardily set ourselves against a holy God. If we were to draw on our knowledge of electrical conduction from elementary school science, pride in effect makes us resistors, not conductors, of God's grace.

Conversely, humble people become conductors of God's grace. So we might say that God gives grace to those who depend on Him; He gives grace to the grateful.

RAISING THE THANKFULNESS BAR

Professing followers of Christ frequently fail to express gratitude to others for acts of kindness done on their behalf. This pervasive spirit of ingratitude is commonplace. I think we overlook the fact that ultimately it is God who gives someone the desire to bless us with, say, a glass of water or a word of encouragement. When we don't pause to thank the person or instrument whom God has sovereignly used to show us His kindness, we most likely are also neglecting to thank God Himself. This grieves the heart of God and is just another variation of failing to acknowledge His goodness toward us. Besides, the attitude of taking God's gifts for granted flippantly presumes upon His grace, which is also not pleasing to God.

There was a time when I rarely thanked God for such things as the availability of hot, running water, anytime of the day; access to good medical care; the security of a house and the warmth and comfort of a cozy bed; the ability to flip a switch and have the light come on; the blessing of food in "my" cupboards and pantries; and the smooth operation of the dishwasher, clothes dryer, and heat furnace. This is no longer the case. What helped promote my heart posture of gratitude was the recognition that all the aforementioned things are luxuries for more than 99 percent of the world's population. Although I'm not close to where I want to be in continually expressing heartfelt thanks to God for His abundant blessings, I'm also not where I used to be.

Charles Spurgeon explained that when a man is underwater, he does not feel the water over his head. Yet, upon coming out, if you were to put a little pail of water on his head, it would become quite a burden for him to carry. Likewise, some of us are swimming in God's mercy. Yet we do not recognize the weight of the glory that God has bestowed upon us. But were we to get out of this ocean of joy, we would begin to appreciate the weight of any one of God's mercies, which now we scarcely notice nor feel grateful for. Without waiting to lose the sense of God's grace and in order that we may know the value of it, let us bless Him who has done such inconceivably great things for us. Let us declare "My soul doth magnify the Lord."[22]

Besides losing the sense of God's grace, ingratitude also short-circuits the flow of joy God desires us to experience. Those who are grateful for the least of God's blessings generally go through life experiencing much joy, while the unthankful person is ever complaining and, not surprisingly, quite often very miserable. For this reason, it is not an overstatement to say that the very quality of our lives is predicated upon how thankful we are.

Even in the midst of difficult experiences, we must choose to remember that God is still good; He still gives us much for which we can be thankful. This is why He commands us to "give thanks in all circumstances" (1 Thessalonians 5:18). This does not mean that we should jump up and down or be exuberant when something painful or heart-wrenching has transpired. God doesn't expect us to deny the devastating situations of life, such as a senseless death, or to pretend that the vicissitudes of life don't cause great distress. But He desires us to be thankful for His unchanging promise that because He is for us and not against us (see Romans 8:31), in His providence all things are ultimately working together for our good as well as for His glory.

22. Charles Spurgeon, *The Fullness of Joy* (New Kensington: Whitaker House, 1997), 145.

TAPPING INTO THE WELL OF DEEPER JOY

This understanding leads to the biblical meaning of joy. Joy is a deep sense of assurance and confidence in God that transcends human understanding. It is not mere happiness, contentment, or overall satisfaction with life; these are predicated upon temporary circumstances. Far deeper than happiness, joy is rooted in the intentional choice to delight in all that God has generously bestowed on us, is currently bestowing on us, and will bestow on us. Many passages in the Bible speak of this deep and abiding joy that God desires us to experience (to name a few, see Nehemiah 8:10; Psalm 51:12, 119:111; John 15:11; 1 Thessalonians 1:19). Therefore, although we may sometimes overlook this truth, being a joyful people is our duty, and the actual pursuit of joy is not optional for a follower of Christ.

GRATITUDE STIMULATES OUR JOY

Earlier in this chapter, I mentioned that God commands us to give Him thanks for our benefit. So is true of the command to be joyful. Scripture is clear that none of God's instructions are given without our benefit (and the benefit of others) in mind. In this case, God's commands to give thanks and be joyful enable us to more actively experience His presence in our daily lives. His abiding joy is a result of His presence. Recall the quote at the beginning of this chapter. God desires that our cup be filled with thanksgiving from the simple recognition that He not only loves us but cares for us in unfathomable ways. He calls us to give thanks because He knows that if the cup of praise and thanksgiving is empty or only half-full, joy cannot overflow and spill into our lives. Joy spilling over becomes even more elusive if the cup isn't being lifted at all. But a cup filled to the brim with praise and thanksgiving will inevitably spill over with joy, even if it is not being lifted. In short, a heightened sense of gratitude to God increases our joy, which brings us to the final spiritual dynamic: *deeper gratitude leads to increased joy.*

As a matter of fact, numerous secular studies have shown that there's a direct or linear relationship between gratitude and joy: the more grateful we are, the more happiness and joy we experience.[23] Among other things, these studies also indicate that practicing gratitude helps people to improve their health, build stronger relationships, and better weather adversity. People who are grateful tend to process their thoughts differently than those who are not. For example, they cultivate the discipline of rejecting thoughts like, *life would be better if only* . . . They're also the proverbial "the glass is half-full" kind of people, who focus more on what they have than on what they do not. Their positive outlook has a beneficial effect on their attitude and, by extension, the joy that they experience. When joy abounds in our hearts, even in the midst of trying circumstances, it can be a wonderful testimony to God's power at work in our lives—our complete trust in Him, no matter what we face, becomes an opportunity for God to be glorified and for others to marvel at the awesome God we serve. Conversely, people who are ungrateful experience less joy and contentedness and very likely all the other aforementioned benefits of practicing gratitude. They also forfeit many an opportunity to declare God's faithfulness and watchful care over their lives.

Many of Christ's followers are going through life with little or no joy at all. Yet it is this deep joy that bolsters us when we walk through the inevitable trials and difficulties of this fallen world. No matter where we may find ourselves, with God's help, each of us can begin to appropriate more and more of His life-giving, soul-stirring joy.

Continually cultivating the habit of expressing heartfelt gratitude for God's goodness also deepens our intimacy with Him. This, in turn,

---

23. "Expanding the Science and Practice of Gratitude," Greater Good Science Center, accessed May 15, 2015, http://greatergood.berkeley.edu/expandinggratitude. "Giving Thanks Can Make You Happier," Harvard Health Publications, accessed May 15, 2015, http://www.health.harvard.edu/healthbeat/giving-thanks-can-make-you-happier.

increases our devotion and commitment. Also recall that gratitude stimulates our fear of God and our desire to love God, both of which are absolutely vital if we are to honor God and build lives of true significance. Like a window, a heart full of gratitude enables us to progressively see more of God's countless blessings and then give Him the thanks and praise that He is rightly due.

As the window through which we see God's goodness is enlarged, thankfulness of heart will gradually replace ingratitude. Most people go through life feeling underappreciated. Together, we can change that! I'm persuaded that, practicing gratitude first toward God and then toward others will truly make a world of difference. It has in my life. Over time, this thankfulness will promote greater humility. As a result of greater humility, we will begin to conduct more of God's grace. Luke 17:12–19 tells the story of ten lepers who are all healed by Jesus. Only one returned to express his thanks. May we live our lives like that one grateful leper and then all the more as we recognize that God has done immeasurably more than simply healed our once sin-diseased hearts— He has given us life everlasting with Him!

Nothing good can ever come out of ingratitude. To be ungrateful is to our peril. Not only does it rob us of joy, it also greatly undermines our spiritual journey. So I want to share these sobering words from John Piper:

> When every human being stands before God on the Day of Judgment, God would not have to use one sentence of Scripture to show us our guilt and the appropriateness of our condemnation. He would need only to ask three questions:
>
> 1. Was it not plain in nature that everything you had was a gift and that you were dependent on your Maker for life and breath and everything?
> 2. Did not the judicial sentiment (the moral faculty that is duly offended when we are mistreated) in your own heart always

hold other people guilty when they lacked the gratitude they should have had in response to a kindness you performed?

3.   Has your life been filled with gratitude and trust toward Me in proportion to My generosity and authority?

Case closed.[24]

Starting today, I encourage you to begin asking your heavenly Father to help you recognize the blessings He sends your way. Then begin thanking Him for each one. Before long, you'll be surprised at the number of His gifts that you've previously taken for granted. In turn, expressing gratitude will become more and more natural. The result is that you'll also begin to experience more and more joy—His deep, abiding joy.

Could it be that the measure of joy we experience in this temporal life will affect the depth of our joy in the next? I think Randy Alcorn provides a relevant thought: "Two jars can both be full, but the one with greater capacity contains more. Likewise, the redeemed of God will be full of joy in Heaven, but some may have more joy because their capacity for joy will be larger . . ."[25]

24. John Piper, *Desiring God* (Sisters: Multnomah Books, 2003), 60–61.

25. Randy Alcorn, *Money, Possessions, and Eternity* (Wheaton: Tyndale House Publishers, Inc., 2003), 126.

CHAPTER 12

·····························

MOTIVATED BY LOVE

There is a hunger in the heart of man that none but God can satisfy,
a vacuum that only God can fill.
—John R. W. Stott

SPIRITUAL THERMOSTAT

In the previous chapter, we learned that the depth of our gratitude to God in response to what He has done for us greatly influences our passion to embrace a life lived for His glory. However, our depth of gratitude does more than just stimulate our passion for God. It actually determines the depth of our love for God—just like it determines the depth of our humility. The root of the matter is that a passionate love for God both anchors and drives our desire to live backward for His good pleasure. Without this intense love, it follows that we absolutely cannot build a truly significant life.

This chapter develops the incredible truth that we *can* learn to love God deeply and to seek Him passionately. But in order to achieve both pursuits, we must have the right motivation.

Heartfelt gratitude affects every facet of our intimacy with God. It is the spiritual thermostat that sets the temperature of our love for God, be it hot, warm, or cold. Essentially, the more grateful we are for what God has done for us, the more strongly we desire to love Him. As our gratitude deepens, so does the intensity of our love.

Luke 7:36–50 gives a touching account that illustrates this biblical truth. Jesus is invited to dinner at the home of a Pharisee. A woman in the town who led a sinful life learned that Jesus was eating at the Pharisee's house and came there with a jar of perfume. Weeping at Jesus's feet, she began to wet his feet with her tears. Then she wiped His feet with her hair, kissed them, and poured the perfume on them. Those present were disgusted by her behavior. In response to their disapproval, Jesus defends, even commends, this woman when He says to the Pharisee: "Do you see this woman? I entered your house; you gave me no water for my feet, but she has wet my feet with her tears and wiped them with her hair. You gave me no kiss, but from the time I came in she has not ceased to kiss my feet. You did not anoint my head with oil, but she has anointed my feet with ointment. Therefore I tell you, *her sins, which are many, are forgiven—for she loved much.* But he who is forgiven little, loves little" (see Luke 7:44–47, emphasis mine). This woman came to Jesus with a repentant heart for her sinful life. Her extraordinary attention to Him was an expression of both her devotion to Jesus and her expectant hope that He would do something for her. If her love for Jesus was this intense even before He forgave her and removed the stain of her numerous sins, it's reasonable to surmise that out of gratitude she loved Him all the more deeply afterward. The facts included in the full account of this story, notwithstanding, draw a clear link between gratitude—for being forgiven of much—and heartfelt love.

Of course the reverse is true: the less grateful we are, the weaker are our affections. If we aren't truly grateful to God for what He has done for us, our desire to love Him will be weak. I invite you to pause and reflect on your relationship with God. There are really only two possible gratitude scenarios: either you recognize that your obedience to God is being strengthened by your heart posture of gratitude or it's the other way around.

According to the Bible, love and obedience go hand in hand. I think we have a hard time *trying* to obey God, rather than just obeying Him, simply because we haven't come to a place of genuine love for Him. Sure, we say that we love Him and we sing that we love Him, yet often He is not uppermost in our affections; we aren't thrilled and overwhelmed by His incomprehensible love for us. As John Piper wisely comments, "The challenge before us then is not merely to do what God says because He is God, but to desire what God says because He is good. The challenge is not merely to pursue righteousness, but to prefer righteousness."[26]

We've previously discussed the unfathomable gift of being adopted into the royal family of the King of the universe. Keeping this in mind, let's purpose to love God more unreservedly; let's resolve to seek Him more wholeheartedly so that He is truly honored in our lives. To do so, we must be keenly aware that, without a heartfelt love for God, we won't desire to earnestly seek after Him and obey Him. Truly, a sincere love for God must always be our primary motivation in seeking Him. My own experience has taught me that any other reason or motivation quickly makes our pursuit of God plain drudgery and unfulfilling.

PASSIONATELY LOVING GOD

To better appreciate the proper motivation for seeking God, it might help to know what it is not. Earlier, we mentioned that servile fear is not the proper motivation for fearing God. This is true because it fosters a dreadful fear that is uncharacteristic of a genuine, loving relationship. In a similar manner, servile love is not the proper motivation for seeking

26. John Piper, "How Dead People Do Battle with Sin," accessed January 11, 2015, http://www.desiringgod.org/resource/how-dead-people-do-battle-with-sin.

God either. It is typically a superficial love that says, "I *must* do this or I *must* do that," out of a sense of mere duty. Loving relationships— be it vertically with God or horizontally with others—should not be primarily characterized by dutiful actions. For instance, I love receiving cards. If my husband were to return from work and surprise me with a romantic card, I'd be delighted by his thoughtfulness. But what if in response to my expression of gratitude he says, "Oh, no big deal, sweetheart; I'm just doing my duty as your husband." I'd be crestfallen. If giving me the card were not a spontaneous and genuine expression of his love, then it's not really a token worth giving. Rather than affirm his love for me, the empty card would devalue my sense of worth to my husband. In a loving relationship, when something isn't done out of an expression of love, gratitude, or admiration, it is merely calculated or dutiful. Rather than build up, this type of action tears down. Instead of giving honor, it dishonors.

If this is true concerning human relationships, what are the implications for our relationship with God? At best, our love toward one another will always be imperfect. However, God alone loves us with the purest form of love there is—He loves us completely, unconditionally, and perfectly. But even though God commands us to love Him, He is not pleasured by our calculated, token expressions of love. Dutiful acts of love (such as ritually attending church with no real desire to be there or begrudgingly giving a tithe or offering to look good to others in church) are actually an affront to God. Like the token card, empty or mechanical actions devalue, not magnify, His worth; they strip God of the supreme honor that He is due. Such an attitude grieves the heart of God who is infinitely worthy of our love and adoration. This is why, although we are commanded to love God, we are also instructed to delight ourselves in Him (see Psalm 37:4). We are to delight in His goodness, grace, forgiveness, mercy, and compassion. We simply cannot delight in something or someone without having our emotions and affections actively engaged.

If you're not convinced of this truth, think of the last time that you were moved to action or an emotional response by something you liked, enjoyed, or appreciated. It may have been the jubilation you felt as your favorite team won in the last split second of a double overtime. Perhaps it was when that unexpected bonus came at just the right time. Put in whatever example you'd like. Did you ponder what your response should be? Was whatever you did or said done apathetically because you *had* to? Or were your actions characterized by great feeling and emotion? Your response was genuine and instinctive, not calculated. In fact, an unemotional response would have been completely unnatural, regardless of the scenario.

If we would truly honor God with our lives, we must learn to love Him from our hearts. The people of Israel often grieved the heart of God by displaying a superficial love toward Him. In response, God lamented, "These people say they are mine. They honor me with their lips, but their hearts are far from me. And their worship of me is nothing but man-made rules learned by rote" (Isaiah 29:13, New Living Translation).

May this not be true of us. Make this commitment to God: I don't want to worship you merely with my lips. I want you to truly be the highest priority in my life—the foremost object of my affections and my heartfelt love. Instead of casually singing worship songs, I want to truly adore you. I desire for your extravagant love toward me to continuously move me to both instinctively and passionately love you.

AN AFFAIR OF THE HEART

Nevertheless, Scripture teaches that it is our duty to love God. But just like falling in love with a human involves a process, so does falling in love with God. If you're already there, that's great! If, on the other hand, you're saying to yourself, "I don't quite have a passionate love for God, but I want to," that's great too! So how do we cultivate this deep and genuine love for God? We find simple clues to answer this question in the verse: "You shall love the Lord your God with all your heart and with all your soul and with all your might" (Deuteronomy 6:5).

Mark 12:30 gives a similar command, "And you shall love the Lord your God with all your heart and with all your soul and with all your mind and with all your strength." The first part of this verse highlights what I've already discussed: though intangible, loving God with our hearts and our souls means engaging Him with feeling or emotion. In contrast, the second part, loving God with all our mind and strength, speaks of a more practical expression of our love. It is also interesting that in Mark 12:30, the command to love God with our heart and our soul precedes the command to love Him with our mind and our strength. I can't help but wonder if there's some significance in the way that these faculties are ordered—because of their outworking in our lives? These attributes seem to logically underscore that our hearts and souls must first be engaged if our minds and will (or strength) are to follow as a matter of course. This order also suggests that we must first know God with our mind before we can love Him with our strength. It's rather difficult to love someone we don't know or barely know. Just like we come to know others by spending time with them, we come to know God by spending time with Him through prayer and in His Word.

It is also noteworthy that loving God *with all our strength* is the very last faculty with which we are commanded to love. Again, this implies that we must love God with our heart before we can ever will to love Him with our strength. The notion of *loving* before *doing* makes plain sense. After all, it's very difficult to will oneself to do something that one does not love. Imagine, for example, running in zero-degree temperature several times a week purely for exercise and recreation if you don't love running. It just isn't going to happen! In general, the only time that we're willing to do something we don't love is because it is expedient for accomplishing something that we do love.

Willing oneself or choosing to do something one doesn't love is very applicable to our relationship with God—we will never gladly obey God until we've come to genuinely love Him. An important point needs to be emphasized here. There are certain times when we may not "feel" like we love God much less desire to love God. During these moments, love will be a choice that we make by faith and God's help. However, this choice or desire to love God would only be stirred in someone who has previously experienced His love, be it on either the giving or receiving end.

The bottom line is that we cannot truly love a God we do not intimately know any more than we can express genuine love to someone unfamiliar to us. Conversely, no matter the inconvenience or sacrifice, we are generally willing to pretty much do anything (hopefully within the confines of God's commands and the laws of the land) for someone we passionately love. Because of our devotion, we take pleasure in displaying frequent and spontaneous demonstrations of our affection. When we truly love God, we'll take delight in adoring Him and showing Him our love.

Of course, at the opposite end are those who don't know God and therefore have no desire to love Him. Then there are those who fall into neither camp, and in Revelations 3:1, God declares: "So, because you are lukewarm, and neither hot nor cold, I will spit you out of my mouth." This stern warning of judgment makes me tremble at the thought of having a weak or conflicted love for God.

A BEATING HEART IS A WALKING HEART

Jesus is clear about our practical response to our love for Him: "If anyone loves me, he will keep my word, and my Father will love him, and we will come to him and make our home with him. Whoever does not love me does not keep my words" (John 14:23–24). Additionally, both John 14:15 and 21 agree, "If you love me, you will keep my commandments."

To love Jesus is to obey Him, just as to not obey Him is to not love Him. The desire to obey is a natural outgrowth of the desire to love—because we love God, we desire to please Him by our obedience. And as our love for God grows, so does our obedience.

Both the desire and ability to obey God is birthed from our love for Him. It can be summed up this way: the heart that *beats* with love for God is the same heart that *walks* in obedience to Him. Hence, a heart beating with love and a heart walking out this love are one and the same. Love for God and obedience to God are two faces of the same coin. You absolutely cannot have one without the other. Therefore, it's impossible to say that we love God, yet not desire to obey what He commands of us. Ultimately, genuine love for God is the only incentive that enables us to bear up under trials and temptations.

Moreover, if we love God for who He is and sincerely desire to pleasure the heart of One so indescribably good to us, then our duty to love becomes a delight. The wonder of God is that He is all that we will ever need.

In his most excellent book, *Desiring God*, John Piper posits this question: "What could God give us to enjoy that would prove Him most loving? There is only one possible answer: Himself! If He withholds himself from our contemplation no matter what else He gives us, He is not loving."[27] The God we are invited to delight in loving is a God who gives us Himself. As we've seen, because God has given us Himself, He has given us *everything!* Why would we not desire to love a God who has been this inconceivably good to us? Maybe we need to earnestly seek to know God better. Perhaps we need to gaze on the incomparable attributes of the Father's radiant glory revealed in Christ (see Hebrews 1:3). We simply cannot adequately admire, praise, adore, and delight in a God whom we have not yet comprehended as being awesome, glorious, praiseworthy, altogether lovely, and beautiful beyond description.

---

27. John Piper, *Desiring God* (Sisters: Multnomah Books, 2003), 47.

CHANGED HEART—CHANGED AFFECTIONS

God desires intimacy with each of His children. This is why He is ever chasing, ever seeking us. In fact, if you are a child of God, you are where you are *only* because He has been relentlessly pursuing you. Sure, you may have been seeking Him too, but recall that it is God who enables us to seek Him in the first place (see Philippians 2:13; John 6:44, 65).

Earlier we saw that our desire to love God is the by-product of our hearts having been regenerated. We learned that regeneration is miraculous and supernatural. The result of regeneration is no less supernatural, namely, a distinctly changed heart—a heart so radically transformed that it wants to truly know God, desires to delight in Him, longs to please Him through obedience, seeks to live for the praise of His great name, and rejoices in fellowship with Him. These are the impulses that motivate us to passionately love God, to worship and adore Him alone! I resonate with John Piper's description of a converted heart:

> In the end, the heart longs not for any of God's good gifts, but for God Himself. To see Him and know Him and be in His presence is the soul's final feast. Beyond this, there is no quest. Words fail. We call it pleasure, joy, delight. But these are weak pointers to the unspeakable experience . . . Happiness in God is the end of all our seeking.[28]

In God's presence we find the fullness of joy (see Psalm 16:11). As we feast on these spiritual delights, we develop an unquenchable desire for more of God's presence. The more time we spend in His presence, the more we are transformed. We begin to make choices and decisions based on a new set of standards. New affections, desires, feelings,

....

28. John Piper, *Desiring God* (Sisters: Multnomah Books, 2003), 87.

goals, disciplines, and interests are all awakened in us. Along with all these comes a deeper motivation to love God as well.

As the pithy saying goes, "The proof is in the pudding!" The proof of our love for God is seen in the things that we seek after and desire. Piper states, "The newness of the creature is that he has a new taste. What was once distasteful or bland is now craved."[29]

The cultivation of this new taste, which makes us crave the things of God, has its genesis in our minds. Our minds exert a powerful influence on the direction of our lives, much more than we even realize. This reality is the focus of the next chapter.

29. Ibid., 72–73.

PRINCIPLE 3

KNOW THE FORCES THAT CAN SUBTLY RUIN OUR LIVES

CHAPTER 13

······························

THE TYRANNY OF THE ROUTINE

There is a great distinction between the urgent and the important. The urgent demands our time, but usually wastes it; the important redeems it, gives it eternal significance.
—Jim Denison

I'm convinced that one of the hardest things in life is to train ourselves to think purposefully whenever our minds are otherwise disengaged. We cannot afford to mentally coast through life . . .

A BUSTLING FORTRESS OF SEVENTY THOUSAND THOUGHTS PER DAY

In this chapter, we'll explore the unequivocal reality that what we think about profoundly determines who we become—for all eternity. In order to live backward, we must take control of our thoughts.

The human mind is a very busy place. Did you know that an average of seventy thousand thoughts run through our minds each day? We're frequently not aware of many of them. It's a paradox, but we tend to not think about what we're thinking about. Thoughts run helter-skelter, because we do not regulate them. We could call this mindless thinking. To make matters worse, the seemingly continuous barrage of incoming media (such as Twitter, Facebook, TV, radio, and the Internet) keeps our minds buzzing with a multitude of different notions. All of these distractions only compound the lack of oversight we give our thoughts. The result is that random ideas infiltrate our minds and subconsciously influence the quality of our inner lives.

Of course, not all thoughts are random and unregulated. Neither do all of them simply pass through our minds. Many stick around and, over time, take up residence. These accepted thoughts or mental occupants can affect us in a myriad of ways. For instance, some make subliminal or subconscious suggestions or appeals. Imagine that the brand of facial product you normally use is out of stock at your local store. You really can't afford to wait, so you decide to buy one of the other available products. But which brand? You're drawn to one in particular as your mind recalls the lively ad that you've seen and heard several times during the past few months. Almost instinctively, your mind is made up as to which new brand you're going to try. At the other end of the spectrum, some mental stimuli enter our minds and instantaneously impose powerful demands. For example, picture yourself at a football game (or your favorite sporting event). Across the jumbo screen comes an ad featuring the "juiciest and most deliciously satisfying burger you've ever enjoyed as a spectator." The burger looks so mouthwatering good that you immediately head to the concession stand to purchase one, even though you're not hungry at all.

Regardless of their frequency, duration, regulation, or whatever effect they have on our minds, thoughts or mental impressions are generally not neutral—they are either beneficial or detrimental to our lives and our spiritual growth.

COMPOUND IGNORANCE

Unless we continually put to death those thoughts that are inconsistent with the character of God, our mind eventually becomes a stronghold of ungodly ideas. We don't even realize how ungodly our minds really are because we don't pay much attention to what we think about in the first place. This pretty much sums up why we are easily blinded to deception, subtle or overt. Also, because we don't pay attention to what we're thinking about, we don't recognize just how blinded we are to the true state of our thought lives. It's like we have compound ignorance: we have not a clue that we are clueless to the fact that our minds are ungodly. This blinder exposes us to even greater deception, which the enemy cleverly uses to make us captive to his will—Satan cleverly uses our very own thoughts to entice and ensnare us.

For this reason, Scripture instructs us to "take every thought captive to obey Christ" (2 Corinthians 10:5). This simply means that if Christ wouldn't think what we're thinking, then neither should we; every thought that is in rebellion to God should be apprehended and submitted to the authority of Christ. The Bible also teaches that the human heart is so deceitful and desperately wicked that we can't know what lurks in our own hearts (see Jeremiah 17:9). Without any help from the enemy, the remnants of sin in our hearts predispose us to deception. Left to ourselves, our hearts will always move us further and further away from the truth. Therefore, we must avoid worldly wisdom that tells us to glibly follow our intuitions. Instead, we should follow our hearts only if they are being instructed by the truths of God's Word.

Our minds are never a vacuum. For instance, something is always on your mind even as you go to bed at night and wake up in the morning. During the day, when you're not engaged in a mental task or your mind is free to wander, where does it go? It definitely goes *somewhere*. Just like each and everything we do is either drawing us toward God or moving us away from Him, we must also recognize that ultimately each of our seventy thousand or so daily thoughts are either moving us closer to or further away from God—treading water is not an option. Like windows into our souls, our thoughts reflect the actual moral and spiritual condition of our heart. Regardless of what we may *believe*, *say*, or *do*, our thoughts are the only accurate index of the true condition of our minds.

Be it consciously or subconsciously, each of our thoughts to some extent influences the overall quality of our thought life, which subsequently affects our mental outlook. Since our minds are the filters through which we view all of life, our seemingly trivial thoughts are potent—they literally dictate the very course of our lives. This is not just a psychological principle, it's a biblical principle: "For as he thinks within himself, so is he" (Proverbs 23:7, New American Standard Bible). And as a man thinks, so he becomes! Just as, physically, we, in a sense, become what we eat, mentally and spiritually we become what we think.

BUILDING BLOCKS

Therefore, our conscious thoughts may be likened to a child's box of building blocks. A child can randomly toss blocks around without building anything useful or constructive, or he can intentionally assemble the blocks to build appealing, imaginative creations. Similarly, we are actually building our lives with the thoughts we think. Like the child, we are either building constructively or idly moving blocks around. The progression of the following wise maxim underscores that what we think determines who we eventually become: "Sow a thought; reap an action. Sow an action; reap a habit. Sow a habit; reap a character. Sow a character; reap a destiny."

And it's based on a biblical principle. Galatians 6:7 states, "Do not be deceived: God is not mocked, for whatever one sows, that will he also reap." We can sow spiritually worthless thoughts and reap the consequences of ungodly thinking. Or we can sow spiritually healthy thoughts that are honoring to God and reap the blessings of godly thinking. Either way, the thoughts we sow will determine the harvest that we reap, not only in this life but in the life hereafter.

Furthermore, many of us go through life largely unaware of the profound reality that our thoughts also have eternal ramifications—they influence our actions, which will eventually determine the sum of our character. Our character will ultimately be the sole measure by which our lives are endowed with eternal significance. We are cautioned, "For we must all appear before the judgment seat of Christ, so that each one may receive what is due *for what he has done in the body, whether good or evil*" (2 Corinthians 5:10; emphasis mine; see also Jeremiah 17:10). I must emphasize that this judgment is not referring to whether a person is saved through faith in Christ, for that cannot be earned; this judgment refers only to our works or what we have done on the earth. Clearly, God will hold each of us responsible for our actions. He has promised that our good works will be rewarded with lasting significance. The inverse of this Scripture is also true: what we choose to not do (or become) in this brief life will result in some measure of insignificance in the life hereafter. So today's thoughts, which speak the quiet language of the heart, are the action words with which our life stories are scripted for all eternity.

What sort of thoughts have you been sowing? What kind of eternal life story have you been building? To one degree or another, each of us has reaped and is still reaping the chaff of ungodly thinking. Thankfully, God mercifully redeems our mistakes and failures so that His purpose for our lives is fulfilled. What's more, He promises to take even what the enemy intended for evil in our lives and transform it into something good (see Genesis 50:20). God is also the God of second—no, millionth—chances. No matter what you have been building with your thoughts thus far, with God's help, you can modify your building strategy and start erecting a mighty spiritual fortress of godly thinking. You can begin to build something constructive, something significant, with your life.

THE EFFECT OF MINDLESS THINKING

Before going further, we first need to switch gears and look at thoughts from an entirely different angle. There's a psychological term called heuristic bias. It means that we tend to think and act in fairly predictable ways. Simply, we like the familiar. It's easy to see how this tendency makes us further predisposed to mindless thinking in our day-to-day routines.

A popular definition of insanity is to do the same thing over and over again and expect different results. I like to think of this tendency as the tyranny of the routine. We're prone to just go through the motions of life. I know because I've been there. However, if we keep doing what we've always done, we'll continue to get what we've always had. So, in what sounds like double-talk, if we want to make some changes in our lives, *we need to make some changes in our lives.* Change begins as we make different choices, and these choices are ultimately a result of how we think.

Since our hearts are naturally deceitful and wicked, left to ourselves, we don't think godly thoughts or act in God-honoring ways. Needless to say, mindless thinking doesn't promote godly thoughts and behaviors; it only compounds ungodly thinking resulting in more ungodly actions. If we're not careful to confront mindless thinking, our thoughts will continue to go unchecked, resulting in even more ungodly thoughts and actions. It is sinking thinking: ungodly thoughts sink us deeper into the morass of sin that erodes our character and destroys our lives. For instance, thinking up one lie leads to telling others, resulting in a greater tendency to tell more (and even more elaborate) lies in the future.

A similar process might happen if someone entertained the idea to view a brief, sexually provocative commercial. In general, doing anything wrong or illegal, even just once, makes it just a little bit easier to do the second time around. So after that one incident, it would increasingly become easier to tune in to such material—and for longer periods at a time. Eventually the person may be unable to resist viewing an entire movie of sexually inappropriate behavior. Over time and left unchecked, this addiction would most likely worsen.

The negative downward progression resulting from an unchecked or unmonitored thought life is applicable across the board. The more we repeat an action that is dishonoring to God, the easier it becomes to subsequently engage in it—to the detriment of our souls. We can be certain that the devil and his minions delight in being our cheerleading team whenever we fall; they take great pleasure in rooting us on in our sins. And it usually works—their schemes serve to fortify sin's grip on us. We end up in a vicious cycle. The more we engage in a sin—intentionally or unintentionally—the easier it becomes to commit that sin again; and as we continue to commit that sin, like bees attracted to flowers, we are drawn to it all the more. For the most part, this tendency explains why addictions (legal and illegal) are so easily formed but very hard to break.

MENTAL RUTS

If we are to honor God with our lives, we must overcome the inertia of ungodly thoughts that lead to ungodly behaviors. We must cultivate the mind of Christ (see 1 Corinthians 2:16). Scripture teaches, "You must have the same attitude that Christ Jesus had" (Philippians 2:5, New Living Translation; see also 1 Corinthians 2:16). We must take to heart, therefore, that our thoughts shape not only our attitude but also our desires, motives, and behavior. In training our minds to be more like Christ's, it's important we understand the actual process whereby wrong thinking leads to more wrong thinking. Sooner or later, predictable thought patterns (heuristic bias) create mental ruts on which incoming stimuli travel and are subsequently processed. If our thoughts are not being conditioned by the precepts of God's Word, we will end up building spiritually unhealthy mental roads. Eventually worldly ideas and ungodly thoughts create huge potholes. These potholes then entice and deceive us, making us more blinded to truth. Just like physical potholes, left to themselves mental potholes only get larger and deeper with time.

In light of this reality, God calls us to dedicate ourselves to the spiritual disciplines that enable us to know and understand His thoughts, desires, and plans for us. Examples of these spiritual disciplines include studying the Bible, meditating or reflecting on its truths day and night (see Joshua 1:8), memorizing Scripture (see Psalm 119:11), fasting (see Matthew 6:16), and praying (see Luke 11:1). Because these disciplines are God's sanctioned means of appropriating His grace and power in our lives, we cannot overcome ungodly thinking nor break the power of sin's empty and deceitful promises by any other means. If we want to truly live in God's grace and allow Him to transform our minds, we must daily give ourselves to these spiritual disciplines, though not necessarily all of them each day.

The bottom line is that the less our minds are being exposed to Scripture, the less our thoughts are rooted in truth. It follows that the less we know God's Word, the fewer opportunities the Holy Spirit has to show us how to apply its enduring truths to our lives. The end result is that we become prone to even greater deception, though not necessarily all of them each day.

The more we are deceived, the more chronic our spiritual blindness becomes. This sets up a vicious circle: the more we neglect the study of God's Word, the worse our spiritual blindness becomes; the more blinded we are, the more susceptible we become to worldly deception and allure. Aggravating this reality are the mindless, spiritually unhealthy thoughts that are still going unchecked, leading to yet greater deception. Hence, we end up with compound or double deception—we become thoroughly blinded by the worldly external stimuli our minds continue to receive.

As a result of our worsening spiritual blindness, our mental filters become more and more ill equipped to process and act upon incoming stimuli in ways that are honoring to God. Clogged with so many ungodly thoughts, our minds gradually become like a malfunctioning traffic signal. Instead of flashing red for ungodly thoughts, our mental filters increasingly flash green. Vice versa, instead of godly thoughts being welcomed by flashing green lights, red lights stop them from influencing how we think. Eventually, the corrupted mental roads we've built invite things such as chronic depression; apathy; uncontrollable anger or temper; food, drug, and sexual addictions; perverted thoughts; and use of pornography. Clearly, failure to sow spiritually healthy seeds robs us of both temporal blessings and eternal treasures.

ROAD UNDER CONSTRUCTION

To confront the tyranny of ungodly thoughts, we must first repair the mental ruts created by mindless thinking that allow random thoughts to negatively shape who we are becoming. Second, we must fill the mental potholes of worldly ideas and ungodly thoughts with the enduring truths of God's Word. In so doing, we'll start to repair our malfunctioning mental filters so that they begin to flash green for godly thoughts and red for ungodly ones. Part and parcel of this mental overhaul is that we must also continuously wage war against sinful thoughts, desires, and motives, choosing instead to fill our minds with thoughts that are true, pure, and admirable (see Proverbs 4:23; Philippians 4:8). Third, we must depend on the Spirit of God to help us apply the scriptural truths we are learning so that our behavior and conduct progressively become more Christlike.

By embracing this threefold process, we can break free from the subtle but treacherous tyranny of ungodly thinking; we can change our thoughts and, subsequently, our actions. As a result of these reciprocal dynamics, each of us can actually begin to weave beauty into the fabric of our lives. Yet this process is only one part of breaking free from ungodly thinking.

GOVERNING OUR THOUGHTS

The other half involves taking continued, active charge of our thoughts in order to foster a more godly thought life. Its foundation is based on a biblical mandate, "Keep your heart with all vigilance, for from it flow the springs of life" (Proverbs 4:23). I like how Randy Alcorn put it:

> If someone wants to pollute water, he pollutes it at its source. If he wants to purify water, he purifies it at its source. Our thoughts are the source of our lives. All our lives flow from our mind, and through the choices we make every day we program our minds, either for godliness or ungodliness . . . The fact is, you and your children will inevitably adopt the morality of the programs, movies, books, magazines, music, Internet sites, and conversations you participate in. GIGO—garbage in, garbage out; godliness in, godliness out. The cognitive is basic to the behavioral—you become what you choose to feed your mind on.[30]

It's so critical we get this truth that garbage in is garbage out. The fact of the matter is that nothing that we see or read just goes into a black hole. Have you at times noticed that long after you've heard a particular song, you continue to hum or sing it in your head, hours

---

30. Randy Alcorn, "Sexual Purity: What You Need To Know," accessed August 18, 2012, http://www.epm.org/resources/1998/Mar/1/sexual-purity-what-you-need-know/.

and sometimes even days later? Images and words are powerful—like thoughts, they, too, imperceptibly shape our hearts, thought patterns, and actions. Godly character is unequivocally our destiny in Christ. We can't feed our minds with worldly or ungodly material—which leads to ungodly thoughts and actions—and then expect godly thinking and living to come forth. Are you eating and digesting the truths of God's Word? Or are you ingesting the world's buffet of self-centered thinking, relativism, humanistic philosophies, and New Age ideas, which all serve to reduce God's moral commands into personal values, opinions, and desires? What you feed your mind will surely birth your choices. Each and every thing you expose your mind to influences your choices, which directly affect your actions, and in turn determines who you eventually become. There is perhaps no better index of what is truly important to us than what we deliberately choose to think about. How we choose to use "our" God-given gifts and invest time greatly factors in; however, if you think about it, it is the way we think or our outlook on life that first shapes these decisions. Although with whom we choose to associate and how we spend money are likewise powerful indicators of what we value, they, too, are strongly determined and influenced by our thoughts. How very true the maxim that our choices eventually make or break us!

Therefore, it's of utmost importance that we start taking constant inventory of what we're thinking about. We must diligently seek God's help to be vigilant about guarding our hearts. (Remember, we are called to guard our hearts for it is the wellspring of our lives.) A simple but very effective way to help this process along is to carefully control our exposure to secular media outlets permeated by worldly values and perspectives that detract us from focusing on what's really important in life. We should also be mindful that numerous studies have shown that the mind cannot distinguish between what's real and what's imagined, so there's no such thing as "Oh, it's just a movie" or

"No big deal, it's just a book."[31] Again, garbage in, garbage out. The following paraphrase of a children's Bible song called "Be Careful Little Eyes What You See" offers a pithy but powerful synopsis of what children and adults alike should be doing if we truly desire to guard our hearts and minds:

Be careful little eyes what you see; be careful little ears what you hear.

Be careful little hands what you do; be careful little feet where you go.

BATTLEFIELD OF THE MIND

We must understand that when we go to the source of our thought lives in order to pursue greater purity of heart, we've chosen to enter into a cosmic spiritual battle. I remember hearing the saying as a child, "The idle mind is the devil's workshop." Make no mistake, mindless, godless thoughts are the devil's cherished tools! The enemy of our souls wants our thoughts to remain, at best, purposeless, and, at worse, vile and corrupt. So as we engage in this battle for our minds, we must heed Scripture, "let the Spirit renew your *thoughts* and *attitudes*" (Ephesians 4:21, New Living Translation; emphasis mine).

As we lean into God to put off carnal thoughts, we gradually begin to think more of his thoughts. God's thoughts are always purposeful. Pregnant with life-giving and life-changing power, they modify our perspective and attitude. As our minds are changed and renewed, so are our behavior and actions (see 2 Corinthians 3:18). As we continue to internalize more of God's thoughts, our values and priorities are transformed, also empowering us to effect godly change in our lives. The resultant change is the practical expression of the biblical mandate to bring forth fruit that proves we have had a change of mind or heart

---

31. David Hamilton, "Visualization Alters the Mind & Body," accessed May 14, 2015, http://drdavidhamilton.com/visualisation-alters-the-brain-body/.

(see Matthew 3:8; Luke 3:8). Over time, the tyranny that mindless, ungodly thoughts wield over us is weakened. This dismantling of our thought life is the first recourse—as well as the antidote—to the subtle yet pervasive tyranny of the routine.

CHOOSE TO DECIDE

It may be tempting to brush aside the importance of guarding what you see and hear in order to govern your thoughts. However, to not make a decision is, by default, to have made a decision. Unless we tenaciously seek to nurture thoughts that are pure, holy, and good, we will default to impure and ungodly ones. The stark reality of neglecting to guard our hearts is this: idleness of thought leads to aimlessness of actions; aimlessness of actions results in the squandering of our time, energies, gifts, and resources, all of which run counter to living backward in order to make our lives count for God's glory. Scripture is abundantly clear that ungodly thoughts arouse ungodly desires that lead us down the path of sin: "But each person is tempted when he is lured and enticed *by his own desire*. Then desire when it has conceived gives birth to sin, and sin when it is fully grown brings forth death" (James 1:14–15; emphasis mine). Therefore, our lack of vigilance toward ungodly thoughts opens us to temptations and sins. What we must understand is that choosing to not guard our hearts amounts to choosing to be vulnerable to sin. And if we were to sin as a result, it would then be deliberate. This attitude is akin to going down a path of our own choosing; it amounts to intentionally going against the directives of the divine GPS. Intentional or rebellious wrong turns that put us on the path of sin result in a failure to live purposefully for God. No matter how much success, popularity, wealth, fame, etc., we achieve as a result of these wrong turns, ultimately they cause us to forfeit a life of true significance.

Take heed that sinful thoughts destroy. Matthew 15:19 attests, "For out of the heart come evil thoughts, murder, adultery, sexual immorality, theft, false witness, slander." (See also Mark 7:20–23.) From the above outcomes, it's clear that sinful thoughts always come with strings attached, affecting not only the offender but potentially many others as well. Just as the birth of a baby always follows conception and never the other way around, so the birth of intentional sin always follows the conception of an ungodly thought. (This is not necessarily the case for sins that we spontaneously commit.) As we experience the fleeting pleasures of purposeful sin, the sinful thought precipitating that particular sin has previously gone through our mind. We must grasp that even ostensibly small thoughts are pregnant with power to produce potentially devastating consequences in our lives. Sexual immorality in all its various forms, lusts of every kind, and chronic lack of integrity all begin as a seemingly small thought. Therefore, to continue in mindless thinking, which leads to ungodly and misdirected actions, is to end up with a wasted life, one that does not honor or glorify God.

Mindless, purposeless, and spiritually misdirected thoughts may be likened to sand, whereas thoughts conditioned by the truth of God's Word may be likened to rocks. I wish to strongly encourage you to not build your brief but oh-so-precious life on sand. Jesus contrasted wise and foolish builders: "Everyone then who hears these words of mine and does them will be like a wise man who built his house on the rock. And the rain fell, and the floods came, and the winds blew and beat on that house, but it did not fall because it had been founded on the rock. And everyone who hears these words of mine and does not do them will be like a foolish man who built his house on the sand. And the rain fell, and the floods came, and the winds blew and beat against that house, and it fell, and great was the fall of it" (Matthew 7:24–27).

THE DELUSION OF SOMEDAY

The last component to confront the tyranny of the routine involves yet another aspect of thinking and acting predictably: we have a propensity for not living life in the present moment. Consider how Blaise Pascal puts it:

> Let each of us examine his thoughts; he will find them wholly concerned with the past or the future. We almost never think of the present, and if we think of it, it is only to see what light it throws on our plans for the future. The present is never our end. The past and the present become our means, the future alone our end. Thus we never actually live, but hope to live, and since we are always planning how to be happy, it is inevitable that we should never be so.[32]

This is so true. We allow the present moment to become our means to the future. As Pascal aptly notes, we then never live. Instead of focusing on what we can do right now in the present, we expend our time and mental energies thinking or worrying about the future. Or we choose to replay our past, often wallowing in regret. We cannot change the past any more than we can exist in the future; with either mind-set, we fail to redeem the time—we fail to live backward.

We must use the currency of the present to purposefully shape our eternal futures. In other words, we must embrace with vigor that how we live each and every day will ultimately determine the sum total of our lives. As we know, the mind-set that every choice and tick in the here and now matters forever is what enables us to maximize the gift of hindsight. Yet we're all too easily inclined to put off the choices we need to make now in order to intentionally shape our future. But if the choices we're making each and every moment will determine our

---

32. Blaise Pascal, *Pensées* (New York: Penguin, 1966), 43.

eternal future, why do we delude ourselves that we can wait and make the important decisions later? Why do we also underestimate what we are capable of doing today, but grossly overestimate what we'll be able to accomplish tomorrow?

I've discovered from personal experience that this pattern of putting off the present results in a state of complacency. Eventually, we come to erroneously view the future not as a place where we are all going, but instead as a place where we may someday arrive. If we're not making wise choices in the present, we are, by default, actually damaging or impoverishing our future. This unshaped or negatively fashioned future will inevitably arrive.

A similar process happens in our relationships with loved ones. If we aren't intentional, we begin to simply go through the motions of being a family. If we desire our relationships to bloom in the future, we must nurture them today. This saying sums it up: "Tend the garden of your children's heart each and every day." This sage advice also applies to marriages. A couple cannot expect to have a healthy, wonderful marriage five years into the future—in fact, it's virtually guaranteed to not happen—if the couple is not intentional about tending and nurturing it today. Yet by default, we tend to undervalue what we don't actively appreciate. People don't plan for cherished relationships with loved ones to wither from neglect; they simply fail to recognize the inertia of their mental ruts.

Never underestimate the importance of encouraging others and telling those you love just how much they matter to you. Husbands and wives should consistently be building one another up, stoking the flames of their marriage so that it burns slow and steady; parents need to continually affirm and encourage the children entrusted to them by God; good friends should show each other how much they care. Don't let precious opportunities to let others know how much you appreciate them as well as why you appreciate them go by. Tell them, each and every chance that you can.

SIXTY MINUTES PER HOUR

We all fall prey to both tyrannies of mindless thinking and routine, which can greatly undermine the abundant and purposeful lives that Jesus Christ died for us to have. Imperceptibly, we become prisoners of the humdrum routines we have created. Often, we become shackled to our stifled dreams. We also fail to pursue our God-given purpose, because, over the course of time, our mindless routines dull the desire to both nurture and pursue our God-given dreams and passions. Before long, these passions become buried beneath our ruts of complacency. Less important priorities displace more important ones, displacing even God's rightful place in our lives. Ultimately, we forfeit growth in godly character.

The plain truth is that we are all embracing the future at a rate of sixty minutes per hour. Whether we go through life mindlessly or intentionally, embrace wise and godly choices, make unwise and ungodly choices, or defer making choices, we will all greet tomorrow and shake hands with the future, provided we are still breathing.

I've heard it said that discipline weighs ounces, but regret weighs tons. Each of us will have to settle accounts with the future regarding the choices and decisions that we've made. We can either pay up front with discipline, or we can pay later on with regret. And it's certain that if we don't discipline ourselves, something or someone else will discipline us. In the interest of our greatest good, we must resolve now to make godly choices and decisions in order to have a fulfilling temporal future that, in turn, will lead to an eternity with fewer regrets and greater reasons to rejoice. We ultimately have nothing to lose and absolutely everything to gain by leveraging the gift of hindsight. So let's do what we may not feel like doing today in order to shape the kind of person we desire to be in the future. Let's honor our God by being who He has called us to be *now*, so that we can be more like He desires us to be tomorrow and for all eternity.

Don't fall for the lies of the enemy or the enchantments of this fleeting life. They both will undermine your spiritual progress and take you away from the path of God's best for your life. Take care that you don't mindlessly put off those things that are of eternal value in favor of short-term goals and pleasures. There's no escaping the truth that in hindsight, our character, or who we eventually become, will show whether we've chosen to pay the price of discipline or the steep price of regret. Most importantly, remember that God will ascribe eternal significance (rewards, treasures, responsibilities), based on how much our earthly lives have come to reflect Christ. By radically confronting both tyrannies of mindless and ungodly thinking, we position our hearts and minds to be more fertile for the things of God. As a result, we will live for what matters to God and bring Him great delight—the heart and soul of living backward.

CHAPTER 14

·······················

RESISTING THE WORLD'S PULL

If you look for truth, you may find comfort in the end: if you look for comfort you will not get either comfort or truth—only soft soap and wishful thinking to begin with and, in the end, despair.

—C. S. Lewis

DON'T FOLLOW THE BLIND

Have you ever used a shopping cart with misaligned wheels that kept the cart from steering straight? Beyond being simply annoying, you have to continually apply pressure in one direction to keep the cart from going in the opposite direction. Otherwise, the cart will determine where you go. The last time this happened, it occurred to me that this is a good illustration of how we must purposefully go in the opposite direction of where the world wants to take us, for it doesn't care one iota about God's glory or who you are becoming. Without a doubt, then, we must resist the pull of the world in order to live backward and delight God's heart.

In 2 Corinthians 4:4, we're told, "the god of this world has blinded the minds of the unbelievers, to keep them from seeing the light of the gospel of the glory of Christ, who is the image of God." People who don't know God are lost simply because they are blind. They cannot see the truth, so they have no desire to walk in it. And unless God supernaturally opens their blind eyes, they will continue to not see. As followers of Christ, we must remember that we are living and working with a large percentage of people who are spiritually blind. They have not received the gift of salvation nor are they blessed to know or understand what God has revealed to us. (This doesn't, however, preclude the likelihood that some of these people will later accept God's free gift.) Neither can they discern the fingerprints of God all around them.

I want to point out two very important points about this reality because they factor heavily into how we engage the world with a Christ-centered perspective. First, we'd hopefully be quite understanding if a blind person were to trip over us or knock something over, because we realize they cannot see. In the same manner, we are called to extend patience, compassion, and grace to those whom we know are spiritually blind. We also should not be surprised when such people engage in behaviors that we know are offensive and dishonoring to God, because their eyes are still darkened to the truth.

Rather than judge or criticize those still dead in sin, we should remember that the only reason we ourselves are no longer spiritually blind is because God has shone the light of the glorious gospel of Christ in our hearts (see 2 Corinthians 4:6). Were it not for grace, we too would still be blind. This awareness should temper our impatience, irritation, anger, and the host of other emotions we tend to display when interacting with those who are spiritually lost. In addition, the knowledge that it's only by God's grace that we're no longer where we used to be should humble us and give us greater compassion for the unsaved.

Secondly, we are called of God to be "a guide to the blind, a light to those who are in darkness" (Romans 2:19). Just as we wouldn't follow someone who is physically blind, we shouldn't pattern our lives after those who are spiritually blind. If God has opened a person's eyes so that he can now see, it would be foolish for such a person to willingly be led astray by someone whom he knows is in spiritual darkness. Both will only end up stumbling and falling. Yet, at times, we're willing to follow those whom we know are spiritually blind, or we let our choices be influenced by those who claim to be able to see, yet whose lives bear little or no evidence that they're walking in the ways of God. By doing either, we easily end up in the ditches of man-centered thinking. Swept up in the rushing current of the secular values of an ungodly world, we start to drown spiritually.

GOING COUNTERCURRENT

Followers of Christ are not called to live for or seek the pleasures of this fallen world. To the contrary, the Bible commands us to "seek first the kingdom of God and his righteousness, and all these things will be added to you" (Matthew 6:33). Yet the things of this world continually beckon to us, constantly enticing us to live for ourselves and to find our pleasure in temporal allurements. Much like having to continually adjust the grocery cart, we must purposefully choose to go countercurrent to the patterns of this world in order to not be conformed by it (see Romans 12:2). If we're not intentional about this, we'll inevitably go with the flow and look and act just like the world around us; we'll behave a lot like gelatin as the world doggedly conforms us to its mold. Indeed, this conformity to the patterns of this world is exactly what is happening to many who claim to be followers of Christ. As a matter of fact, a recent survey done by the Barna Group indicates that there's essentially no qualitative difference between a nonbeliever and a follower of Christ.[33] What a blight on our witness and testimony as Christ's disciples.

The Bible emphatically teaches that followers of Christ are in this world but not of this world (see John 17:14). According to Matthew 7:16, true followers should be known by their fruit. That we should be distinctly different from the world is a given—different in terms of our priorities, our values, our goals, and how we invest our time. In short, we should stand out because of God's very *presence* in us—the more we grow in Him, the more we should shine the light of His presence in this fallen, dark, and hopeless world. The King James translation of 1 Peter 2:9 refers to God's children as a peculiar people. Yes, we should look and act peculiar! People should never have to guess whether we're followers of Christ. When we live our lives according to the precepts of God's Word, virtually every aspect of our lives should be starkly different than those who are of this world. Christ indeed will be front and center, and we'll desire for all that we say and do to point to Him, whenever and wherever. For certain, we will have our share of trials, struggles, challenges, ridicule, and even persecution, yet Jesus reassures us, "I have said these things to you, that in me you may have peace. In the world you will have tribulation. But take heart; I have overcome the world" (John 16:33).

SHEEP CAN EASILY GET TURNED AROUND

Jesus also has not called us to live in a comfortable Christian bubble. If we settle for making happiness, personal comfort, and the pursuit of worldly pleasures our aim in life, we will continue to distance ourselves from a vibrant relationship with God and reap the negative consequences of ungodly choices. The more we get turned around by

33. David Kinnaman, "Christians: More Like Jesus or Pharisees?," Barna Group, accessed October 12, 2013, https://www.barna.org/barna-update/faith-spirituality/611-christians-more-like-jesus-or-pharisees#.VMMf6kfF9qo.

the patterns of this world, the more we stumble, fall, and lose our way. It won't be long before we have wandered far away from the sheepfold of God. But to go outside the boundaries of the fold is tantamount to not having the rod and staff of the Good Shepherd guiding us. This is like purposefully unplugging the divine GPS. Jesus said, "My sheep hear my voice, and I know them, and they follow me" (John 10:27). It becomes increasingly difficult to hear the voice of our Shepherd the further away we've strayed. Without His guidance and protection, we easily fall for the teachings of "false prophets, who come to you in sheep's clothing but inwardly are ravenous wolves" (Matthew 7:15). These false teachers skillfully twist the truth of God's Word and peddle deception to the spiritually naïve who are unable to recognize half truths and lies for what they really are.

We also become more vulnerable to Satan, whom the Bible describes as a roaring lion who walks about seeking whom he may devour (1 Peter 5:8). Satan is in every sense the archenemy of our souls. Because he wants nothing more than to pounce on us and rip our lives apart, he takes great delight in us being far away from the safety of the sheepfold. He knows that the further away we are from God's path, the more vulnerable we are to his lies and the more easily we fall prey to his cunning and deceit. The more the enemy attacks us, the more our lives become characterized by despair, hopelessness, failure, and defeat. Of course, we then further miss out on the full life that Jesus Christ died for us to have. For these reasons, every sincere follower of Christ must heed the biblical teaching to not forsake the fellowship of others in the faith (see Hebrews 10:25).

SOMETHING'S MISSING

Many of us are missing out on the abundant life. We lack joy, peace, direction, contentment, and a genuine sense of purpose. We worry rather than trust God with the details of "our" lives and the lives of "our" families, glossing over the reality that choosing to worry is choosing to not trust God. Many of us are also experiencing a gnawing feeling that our lives aren't quite measuring up to all that God desires for us. Deep down in our hearts, we yearn for so much more. We know that God is for us (see Romans 8:31) and that He desires us to have an abundance of His love, joy, peace—indeed all His promised blessings—yet these spiritual treasures elude us.

Clearly, something is wrong. It seems a significant part of this challenge is that the world's system has usurped the place of God's Word in our lives. I remember when the enemy enticed me with its glamorous lies and empty promises. I bought into some of them simply because I didn't fully know or understand God's heart for many areas of my life.

Our preoccupation with the things of this life usurps the zeal that we should have for God. Yet God is ever faithful to us. This is why He lovingly commands, "Buy truth, and do not sell it; buy wisdom, instruction, and understanding" (Proverbs 23:23). If we don't buy the truth, we'll for certain end up buying the lies of the enemy and the world instead. Both seduce us to compromise our fellowship with God, which leads us down the path of spiritual ruin. We do well to remember that temptations wield power by enticing us to believe that we'll be happier by giving in. It is only by finding a superior satisfaction in God that we're able to break free from the allure of sin. I like how John Piper poignantly puts this idea: "If my thirst for joy and meaning and passion are satisfied by the presence and promises of Christ, the power of sin is broken. We do not yield to the offer of sandwich meat when we can see the steak sizzling on the grill."[34]

---

34. John Piper, "How Dead People Do Battle with Sin," accessed January 11, 2015, http://www.desiringgod.org/resource/how-dead-people-do-battle-with-sin.

YOU DON'T NEED IT!

As part of my due diligence in writing this book, I paid attention to some of the commercials coming across the airwaves. Without question, consumerism deliberately preys on unsuspecting Americans. Not only am I both amazed and flabbergasted that people are falling for these outrageously inflated ads, I've become incensed with what I hope is a righteous anger. Commercials are literally destroying the health, vitality, and the overall well-being of the American people. Feeding the desire to have more, bigger, and better, they continually promote materialism and self-indulgence. Though some are beneficial, the vast majority of ads entice and deceive us while exploiting our sinful cravings. By appealing to the carnal desires lurking in our hearts, they set afire our lusts and passions, over time enslaving us.

Manufacturers use commercials to glibly persuade us that their products are good, always serve our best interest, and are essential to our lives. Yet they know full well that these things can't truly satisfy us. In fact, manufacturers are very much aware that we think and act in fairly predictable ways, so they exploit our natural tendencies, persuading us that their products will satisfy our unmet needs and wants. They seduce us to believe, for example, that a new hair color, a redecorated kitchen, a relationship, or a twenty-pound weight loss can actually fill the hole in our hearts that only God can fill. Take a look at how the following commercials appeal to our self-centeredness:

Credit card commercial: "Reflect your success!"—*More consumer debt from potential credit card misuse doesn't reflect success.*

Phone commercial: "The meaning of life is to stay in touch with your friends!"—*Is the meaning of life this shallow?*

Home-building supply store: "Improve your life!"—*Will remodeling a kitchen really improve your life? With this appeal, many of us may be tempted to spend more time improving the homes we live in than actually improving our lives. Someday, every material thing will be reduced to rubble. Our lives are eternal.*

Motorcycle commercial: "You only get one shot; I want to leave this life exhausted."—*That's fine, but at the end of one's life, is leaving exhausted what truly matters?*

We fall for this sort of twisted, misleading consumer advice each and every day. We casually allow our hearts and minds to be aroused by the very stimuli, which, in the long run, often proves to be, at best, disadvantageous and, at worse, pernicious to our souls. We must come to grips that whenever we turn on the TV set, we risk being influenced and lured by its enticing appeals. We can ill afford to willingly allow ourselves to be mastered in this way. Of course, I'm not suggesting that we never watch television. I am saying that as discussed in the previous chapter, we must vigilantly guard what we allow into our hearts and minds.

BATTLE FOR OUR SOULS

Each and every day, the world and the enemy are waging a direct and strategic campaign against us. This battle of unparalleled proportion is for nothing less than the lives and souls of not only ourselves but also those we love. The stakes are only getting higher as the world becomes more evil. In fact, we live in an age when marriage infidelity, pornography, drug abuse and addictions, materialism, greed, superstition rooted in astrology and the New Age movement, sorcery, homosexuality, falsehood, and rebellion against authority abound. As should be expected, the casualties are indeed many. Marriages are stagnant. Dads are absent. Divorce rates continue to rise. Lives are falling apart. And families are unraveling. Followers of Christ are not exempt from these dismal statistics; indeed, many of us are not walking through life victoriously.

We are thirsty and hungry. Even manufacturers realize this. Thankfully, God has given us another incredible invitation: "Come, everyone who thirsts, come to the waters; and he who has no money, come, buy and eat! Come, buy wine and milk without money and without price. Why do you spend your money for that which is not bread, and your labor for that which does not satisfy? Listen diligently to me, and eat what is good, and delight yourselves in rich food. Incline your ear, and come to me; hear, that your soul may live" (Isaiah 55:1–3).

We don't have to scrounge for crumbs because our gracious heavenly Father has prepared a lavish dinner for us. We have all been given a blood-bought right to delight in the richest of fare as we look to God as the source for all that we need. Buying milk and honey is part and parcel of standing at the crossroads and asking for the good way. It is by feasting on the delights of God alone that we are empowered to intentionally swim against the rapids of deception and currents of worldly enticements that are ever seeking to pull us under. We can't let up on pushing against the flow of the bankrupt culture of this world—or we'll end up in the evil and corrupt places where it flows. God's truth alone sets us free from the bait of the enemy, the deceitfulness of this world, and the bondage of fleshly desires. If we are to effectively launch counterattacks against these enemies of our souls, we must have more of the Lord's presence and power.

PRINCIPLE 4

....

GROW IN CONFORMITY TO CHRIST

CHAPTER 15

······················

BECOMING FILLED WITH MORE OF GOD

If my life is fruitless, it doesn't matter who
praises me, and if my life is fruitful, it doesn't
matter who criticizes me.
—John Bunyan

SEEING GOD

According to C. S. Lewis, if you want to know God, "the instrument
through which you see God is your whole self. And if a man's self is
not kept clean and bright, his glimpse of God will be blurred—like the
moon seen through a dirty telescope."[35] If we are to see and know God,
we must be willing for God to make our instruments a little cleaner . . .
a little brighter. Therefore, God desires us to be progressively emptied
of ourselves so that we may be increasingly filled with more of Christ.
In other words, we must yield our hearts and our lives to Christ—
not attempting to improve ourselves in our own strength but, rather,
exchanging our lives for His. In the process, we discover our utter inef-
fectiveness and powerlessness if His life isn't flowing in and through us.

······················

35. C. S. Lewis, *Mere Christianity* (New York: HarperCollins, 2003), 164.

This progressive transformation is the heartbeat of living backward. Scripture refers to the process as sanctification. I briefly discussed this topic in Chapter 7. Here I'll develop it more fully. Sanctification begins the moment we genuinely place our trust in Christ as our Savior. It is accomplished by the work of the Spirit of God in our hearts. Picture a glass of water darkly tainted with ink gradually becoming more and more diluted with clear water. This is a picture of what happens as God's presence in us progressively displaces self-love and fleshly passions. Because remnants of corruption still war against our spirit even though our old life is dead (see Romans 7:22–23; Galatians 5:17), the ink of our fleshly desires will not be fully displaced until Christ either calls us home or returns for us.

Remember God's grace comprises two key biblical truths: First, the gift of salvation is completely God's work effected on our behalf—there is *absolutely nothing* we can do to earn favor or right standing with God (see Ephesians 2:5; 8–9). Second, although we are *absolutely powerless* to change ourselves with our own strength, God didn't save us to leave us just as we were. He has saved us that we may be set apart for His purposes, which most fundamentally means being progressively conformed to the nature of Christ.

But before discussing the sanctification process, it's important that we have a rudimentary understanding of who the Holy Spirit is. There was a point in my own spiritual journey when I lacked this understanding and it hindered me from walking in more of the fullness of Christ. For example, I knew of the Holy Spirit, but my understanding of Him was very limited. I knew that He inspired the writing of Scripture and played a vital role in the work of creation, but in reality I had generally conceptualized Him to be more of a something than a person. I didn't grasp that He was the person of the Trinity who awakens faith in us by manifesting the beauty and trustworthiness of Christ. I didn't understand that He is just as much God as is God the Father and God the Son. This is to say, He possesses infinite wisdom, intelligence, and ingenuity, and because He has emotions and feelings, He can be pleasured or grieved. Additionally, I had no idea of His ministry in the lives of disciples. He convicts us of sin and subsequently opens our eyes to the truths in God's Word, His indwelling presence empowers us to access God's grace, love, and mercy, and His inscrutable workings in our hearts and minds transform us from glory to glory so that we live for God—imitating Him, experiencing victory over sin and the enemy, walking in boldness, and bearing fruit that will last (see Ephesians 5:1; 2 Corinthians 3:12; 1 Corinthians 15:7; Galatians 5:22–23; John 15:16). About twelve years ago, I came to intimately know the Holy Spirit, and it is an understatement to say that my life and relationship with Christ have never again been the same.

WE PLANT; GOD BRINGS THE SUNSHINE

From personal experience, I know that sanctification can be a difficult concept to grasp. Although the Bible commands us to pursue our own sanctification, it also teaches that we can do so only in dependence on the Holy Spirit. Because sanctification involves our cooperation with the Holy Spirit, it's easy to misunderstand how the two roles work in tandem with one another.

Here's an illustration of our role and the Holy Spirit's role in sanctifying us. (I wish to give credit to Jerry Bridges here. In his excellent book, *The Discipline of Grace*, he uses a similar analogy, which helped to crystallize this dynamic for me.) First, I want to emphasize that God once and for all justifies us by faith alone—apart from works. However, this faith must also bring forth the fruit of good works in us or else it is dead (see James 2:14–18).

Imagine that someone wants daffodils in her front yard. During the fall, she must cultivate the soil, plant the seeds, add fertilizer, and regularly water the soil. She knows that if she doesn't diligently fulfill these activities, there will be no daffodils adorning her front porch in the spring. Nevertheless, she realizes that she must depend on God to provide the sunshine for the seeds to germinate and bloom. She is clear as to how her role works in tandem with God's: while she understands that she cannot do what only God can do, she also recognizes that God will not do what she herself must do.

Our sanctification is very similar. While there's self-sufficiency, self-pride, self-love, self-reliance, and self-assurance, there's no such thing as self-sanctification. We absolutely cannot attain any degree of holiness without the power of the Holy Spirit effectually at work in us. But just as certain, we cannot attain it without any effort on our part. As I've mentioned, we often confuse our role and responsibilities with God's. Part of the reason is that we can be plain indolent— we want God to do for us what He has called us to do for ourselves. For example, we may pray for deliverance from a besetting sin, even though we aren't willing to memorize a Scripture verse pertaining to the specific sin that the Holy Spirit can bring to our recollection at a vulnerable moment. Needless to say, the Holy Spirit will not do the work of Scripture memorization for us. However, when we do our part, He does His mysterious work in our hearts, pulling out a wrong belief here, illumining a truth there.

I like how C. S. Lewis described God's active involvement in our transformation: "[We do] not think God will love us because we are good, but that God will make us good because He loves us; just as the roof of a greenhouse does not attract the sun because it is bright, but becomes bright because the sun shines on it."[36]

GETTING OFF THE PERFORMANCE TREADMILL

Understanding the above quote is both freeing and motivating. When we understand that God loves us despite our sins, we can stop trying to perform to earn His love and instead pursue true growth in holiness. We do so being confident that God in His omniscience has seen us

36. C. S. Lewis, *Mere Christianity* (New York: HarperCollins, 2003), 63.

at our absolute worst yet He chooses to love us unconditionally and perfectly anyway. Hence, a surrendered heart is the only acceptable offering we can bring to God. In fact, if our pursuit of holiness is not motivated by an ever-increasing understanding of God's unmerited goodness toward us and His complete acceptance of us, it will quickly degenerate into a burdensome activity. When we strive to be pleasing to God in our own strength, it will always leave us frustrated and discouraged because it's a self-centered pursuit that God will never honor. Trust me, I've tried.

However, when we look to God for strength, He delights to help us. God wants to empower us to progressively walk out the truth that, as our Lord and King, Christ is infinitely worthy of our obedience—not partial or delayed obedience but immediate, wholehearted obedience. In the remainder of this chapter, I'll share anecdotal stories that highlight nuggets of truth I've discovered in my own pursuit of holiness.

BUT . . . THE TREE IS IN THE WAY

God uses various things to deepen our understanding of spiritual truths. Several years ago, God impressed upon me the following mental picture: A very large tree is situated just a few feet away from a window. Since the tree is the same height as the window, it's all you see when you look out. The tree represents our self-absorption, because it obscures so much of our outlook on life. We could say that when we peer through the window, all we see is ourselves: we're mostly concerned about our opinion, how we feel others should treat us, what we selfishly desire, or how something wasn't done just the way we wanted. Yet, as difficult as it might be for us to accept, life isn't really about us getting our way. If we are to learn to view life through God's eyes, He needs to set us right.

In sanctifying us, God's work in our hearts is akin to chopping down the tree of our self-love. I know experientially that the more our tree of self-love is cut down to size, the more clearly we see ourselves in proper relation to God: He is God and we are his creation. We live not for ourselves but for what God our Father wants and desires. The less self-absorbed we become, the better our view beyond the window— more of God.

Over time, though we are still tempted to focus on ourselves, we no longer want to gratify our self-love. Eventually, we come to a place where we desire to see even more of God and to view life more from His perspective. The Holy Spirit also helps us to see the true condition of our hearts, and we come to loathe the sins that we see in our lives. This results in genuine brokenness and repentance. It is this truthfulness and brokenness before God that ushers in greater holiness in our lives. Through this refining process, God is able to progressively transform us from the inside out.

BROKEN BUT BEAUTIFUL

Paradoxically, we become more beautiful in God's sight when we see the sins that we were previously blinded to. It follows that until our eyes are opened to our sins, we won't seek change. Hence, the uncovering of sin should promote our continued growth in holiness, making us more and more pleasing to God.

I WANT TO BE A SLAVE!

As we seek Christlikeness, it helps to recognize that every virtue in the spirit has a corresponding vice in the flesh. For example, humility and faith are virtues, whereas pride and disbelief in God are respective vices. Not properly channeled, even a virtue can become a vice, as in taking great care to make plans resulting in "paralysis of analysis" that keeps one from fulfilling a God-given task. Vices are sins, and sin is a cruel slave master (see John 8:4). Although we may feel free when we gratify our sinful desires, in reality we are really slaves. Slaves are anything but free. I like how A. W. Tozer puts it:

> We must of necessity be servant to someone, either to God or to sin. The sinner prides himself on his independence, completely overlooking the fact that he is the weak slave of the sins that rule his members. However, the man who surrenders to Christ exchanges a cruel slave driver for a kind and gentle Master whose yoke is easy and whose burden is light.[37]

We are engaged in a spiritual battle for our surrender, obedience, and worship. Jesus is the infinitely benevolent master who draws and binds our hearts with cords of love. As we've learned, we are truly free only when we become fully committed to Jesus. Being His slave is pleasant. On the contrary, Satan is a cruel slave master who draws us with chains of force and compulsion. Jesus always separates what we do from who we are. Satan does the exact opposite, deceiving us to believe that who we are is based on what we do. Whose slave will you choose to be?

COMPOUND LOVE

The only slave master worse than Satan is our own self-love. As a famous Pogo comic strip goes, "We have met the enemy and he is us."[38] Indeed, the whispers of self-love can be even more powerful than the voice of the enemy. It is blind and hypocritical—what we hate in our own selves is the very thing that we tend to most hate in others. What a double standard.

---

37. A. W. Tozer, *The Pursuit of God* (Camp Hill: Christian Publications, Inc., 1993), 98.

38. Walt Kelly, "This Day in Quotes," accessed January 23, 2015, http://www.thisdayinquotes.com/2011/04/we-have-met-enemy-and-he-is-us.html.

I've now come to realize that I didn't start to truly love and live until I began to hate my selfishness, sin, and ugly behaviors. I didn't make spiritual progress until I had begun to fully embrace that all the emotional pain God had allowed (and was allowing) in my life was to help bring me to that place where I hated myself for caring so excessively about myself. I came to hate that I was so self-centered when things didn't go the way I wanted them to and that my perspective on an issue often tended to exclude the perspectives of others. In the process of God changing my heart, I've learned that I cannot be free to love others the way He intends me to until I loathe and cease to nurture my self-love.

The longer I live, the more I realize that the secret to a joy-filled and contented life is getting myself (or my self-love) out of the way and denying myself the presumed right to defend my self-love in my interactions with others. I am persuaded that the preponderance of our woes in life are primarily rooted in two things: first, our robust self-love and, second, our vehement response to unfulfilled or unmet desires.

Pause for a moment and think about the most recent conflict you've experienced. If you were to simply remove what *you* personally and adamantly wanted or desired out of the picture, could you have potentially spared yourself much talking and arguing and heartache? Would the conflict even have ensued or escalated the way it did? Again and again I see this reality being played out in my life: the more I squelch the persistent desire of my self-love to express itself, the happier, more joyful, and more contented I generally tend to be. I also find myself less irritated, less angry, and less disappointed with those I interact with. I've now come to understand that this death to self-love is integral to the biblical command to die to self. It is also part and parcel of the admonition to make no provision for the flesh (see Romans 13:14).

Finally, we will never know the evil in our hearts until we desire to seek the Lord's help to purify us (Psalm 139:23–24). Until the desire to be holy is formed in our hearts, we will continue to think more highly of ourselves than we should. In fact, the reason people think of themselves as "good" is that they simply have not seen or comprehended the evil in their own hearts. Therefore, we are growing in holiness the more we see and confront the remnants of sin still in our hearts.

MY, HOW YOU'VE GROWN!

Watching the sons and daughter God has entrusted to me get older, it occurred to me that their growth spurts are akin to spiritual growth. Being around them all the time, it's hard to see the actual growth. But when they have grown an inch or two, I suddenly notice it. Something very similar happens with our sanctification. Though often imperceptible to us, God is steadily working on our hearts. Exactly how, we don't always see, have awareness of, or even understand. When we feel as though we're making little progress, we just may be growing deep roots in Christ. If you've ever experienced a time when you surprised yourself with a more godly response than you'd previously demonstrated, then you know exactly what I mean.

I BAKED A CAKE FOR YOU!

Imagine you're a parent returning from work. Greeting you at the door is your smiling ten-year-old daughter. After a great big hug, she excitedly tells you she's baked a cake for you just because she loves you. Touched by her sweet and thoughtful gesture, you plant a warm kiss on her forehead. Placing her hand in yours, she walks you into the kitchen where you are momentarily taken aback by what you see. It's a mess: in addition to several dirty bowls and measuring cups in the sink, there's globs of cake batter on the counters, flour strewn all over the floor, and the splatter of egg yolk on the refrigerator door. What is your response? Would you choose to focus on the messy kitchen, or would you delight in the lopsided cake perched on the island, a tender expression of your daughter's sincere desire to pleasure your heart? There was a time when I would have been tempted to comment on the messy kitchen before expressing gratitude for the cake. But God's sanctifying work is changing me.

In 1 Samuel 15:22, it states that God desires our obedience rather than our sacrifice. God our Father views our earnest attempts to honor Him with our lives like a parent seeing a cake and a messy kitchen. When we mess up, God looks primarily at our motives. If we were sincerely seeking to be obedient, He's less focused on the mistakes we've made. Rather, He looks beyond the mess and delights in our heart posture to please Him.

This simple truth was of great help to me during a period of my life when I was tempted to get stuck in feelings of guilt even after I had confessed my sins and *knew* that God had forgiven me. As I mentioned earlier, this is a common ploy of the enemy. When the Holy Spirit pricks our conscience, it is always accompanied by an awareness that in Christ, God always gives us hope for change. On the contrary, condemnation from the enemy is always accompanied by nagging feelings of failure and defeat. Thankfully, God assures us that if we confess our sins, He is faithful to forgive us and cleanse us from all unrighteousness (see 1 John 1:9).

The cake illustration above highlights another truth: our heavenly Father takes notice of each and every time we set our hearts to please Him—just like earthly parents take joy in their child's efforts to please. We need make only one tiny step in His direction, and He reaches toward us, embracing us in His love. I've discovered a powerful truth—those who daily pursue holiness also experience the deepest joy, for they are continually wrapped in the warmth of their Father's embrace. Yet we must bear in mind that doing the right thing for the wrong reason or the wrong thing for the right reason to "please" God is neither virtuous nor character building. In fact, it ultimately is disobedience. Therefore, no matter how "good" a pursuit or desire may be or seem to be, if we do anything with the knowledge that it is sin, our Father is not pleased (see James 4:17).

FLYING AN AIRPLANE

Sanctification is like flying an airplane that we will never land, no matter how close we may come to approaching the runway. Sometimes it feels like we're ascending or making progress in our spiritual growth, while other times it feels like we're descending. The flight may at times be smooth, but, invariably, we will hit turbulence. Similar to a pilot, we need to make flight adjustments. For accurate information, a pilot needs to be in constant communication with the control tower. God is our perfectly trustworthy air traffic controller. Better yet, the sovereign God of Heaven and earth *is* the control tower. God has promised to give us all the guidance and direction that we need as we diligently seek Him. After all, He is infinitely aware of our air space, fully cognizant of the minutest detail of our flight, and has expert knowledge about each and every weather condition that we will ever face. We can trust Him to show us our flight path. We can also have complete confidence that He will never abandon us in midair.

God's work in us won't be completed on earth. We are spirits who possess bodies, not bodies who possess spirits. My husband, a former computer software engineer, likes to refer to the current bodies that we inhabit as version 1.0. We will not be made perfect in these earthen shells. But our mortal bodies, which are "sown in dishonor," will some-day be "raised in glory" (1 Corinthians 15:43) to a 2.0 version! Some great and glorious day, our plane will touch down on Heaven's celestial runway. Upon our wondrous disembarking, we'll see our magnificent Savior face-to-face and join Him to live forever and ever with God!

SHOVELING SNOW

Several winters ago, we got fourteen inches of snow in a twenty-four-hour period. Since we don't have a snow blower, we removed the snow the good old-fashioned way—with shovels. After hours and hours of shoveling, we still had so much snow to remove. It suddenly occurred to me that shoveling fourteen inches of snow from a 250-foot-long driveway is a lot like sanctification. The more I shoveled, the more I realized just how much snow remained.

GOD'S TOOLS OF REFINEMENT

Families are one of God's finest tools, providing countless opportunities for the life of Christ to flow through us to others. God has placed us in families to refine us, test us, frustrate us, challenge us, mature us, anger us, and try our patience—so that we may be continually challenged to bring forth the fruit of the Spirit: love, joy, peace, patience, kindness, goodness, faithfulness, gentleness, and self-control (see Galatians 5:22–23). God calls us to do the everyday family things as though they were great—whether it's washing dishes, folding clothes, saying a kind word when we'd rather say something unloving, listening to what's in a child's heart despite being exhausted, or being gracious when we just don't feel like it. Time and again, God has used my family to help me become more loving and patient in my interactions not only with them but also with others.

We need to thank God for the people who sometimes bring out the worst in us. Someday we just might have to thank them for shining us up and making us more like Christ. No matter what we may think of others or how much we allow their behavior to negatively influence how we feel, the fact remains that absolutely no one has offended us to the extent that we have sinned against and offended God.

LITTLE THINGS

Indeed, God calls us to great work in unexpected ways. Luke 16:10 plainly teaches, "Whoever can be trusted with very little can also be trusted with much." Because little things greatly matter to God, He desires us to be obedient in the littlest of things. Too often, however, we tend to concern ourselves with the big things and allow the "little" things to go unnoticed or undone. God desires our obedience in the big and little things alike because our obedience in even the littlest of things is an accurate index of our heart posture to be submitted to God in everything. Remember the Pharisees who believed they were worshiping God by their big acts of obedience like fasting and paying their tithes? Yet Jesus sternly rebuked them when He said, "Woe to you, scribes and Pharisees, hypocrites! For you tithe mint and dill and cumin, and have neglected the *weightier matters* of the law: justice and mercy and faithfulness. These you ought to have done, without neglecting the others" (Matthew 23:23; emphasis mine; see also Luke 11:42). The fact that this teaching is mentioned twice in the Gospels underscores just how serious little things matter to God. God can and desires to use the littlest things for His glory.

Sometimes I unwittingly act just like the Pharisees. Many of us do. The things we consider important often matter little if at all to God, and the things we casually brush aside are often the very things that God considers weighty. Some of us have excelled at big things like going to church, participating in a Bible study, or spearheading a church event or committee, but have frequently fallen down in what we see as little things. So we casually neglect what we know *to do.* For example, someone may commit to show up at a meeting fifteen minutes early to get the coffee brewing before others arrive but, for a number of frivolous reasons, fail to follow through. Similarly, we tend to disregard the important things in terms of how God has called us *to be.* For instance, we sometimes fail to show even the smallest act of mercy to a friend or loved one by being critical, sarcastic, or judgmental. Both of these attitudes contradict God's desire for us to act justly and to love mercy (see Micah 6:8). In a different vein, many of us don't adhere to the posted speed limit because we believe it's just not a big deal. Yet Scripture clearly instructs us to be subject to the governing authorities (Acts 13:1–4). Since most of us drive each day, a practical way to start demonstrating faithfulness in the little things is choosing to habitually drive the posted speed limit. God delights to honor our obedience.

GREATER OBEDIENCE RESULTS IN LESS CHASTENING

An earthly parent who is loving and fair would never dole out a negative consequence for no reason at all—discipline is always administered as a corrective measure for a child's misbehavior. As the child progressively learns to conform his behavior to the parent's rules or expectations, he requires less and less corrective discipline. In the same way, God disciplines us for our own good, "that we may share his holiness" (Hebrews 12:10). As our behavior becomes more conformed to the nature of Jesus in a specific area, God doesn't need to chasten or correct us as often as He previously would have had. There's more. I've learned that Satan recoils out of our lives when we take the very things he desires to destroy us—like a betrayal, difficult boss, or cantankerous coworker—and use them to become more like Christ.

BEING LED BY THE SPIRIT

God created us for fellowship with Him, and fellowship involves communication. Yet I've heard many Christians say they don't know how to hear from God. God is always communicating with us through His Spirit.

If we're seeking to follow Christ, our fleshly desires are constantly warring against our spirit. Galatians 5:17 states, "For the flesh desires what is contrary to the Spirit, and the Spirit what is contrary to the flesh. They are in conflict with each other, so that you are not to do whatever you want." We are continually confronted with situations where we have to either deny our flesh what it wants or give in to it and sin. At any given moment, when we sense our fleshly nature rising up in us, the opposite of what it wants is generally what God desires.

Each and every time that our flesh bristles for not getting its way, God is indirectly communicating with us, reminding us not to be slaves to the sinful desires of our flesh but to yield instead to His Spirit in us (see Romans 13:14). The issue then is not that we don't hear from God or that we don't know how to hear from Him. Instead: Are we willing to obey what He communicates to us? Will we choose to gratify our flesh or obey the Spirit of God?

Although the practical application may not be easy, the concept itself is quite simple. The Bible teaches that "all who are led by the Spirit of God are sons of God" (Romans 8:14). If we're soft and supple instead of stubborn and rebellious, the Holy Spirit is always pricking our consciences and guiding us toward truth so that we don't go the way of our flesh. Therefore, being led by the Spirit primarily means that He empowers us to put to death our known sins and to not gratify the lusts of our flesh—it's not just a rapturous emotional state, vision, or inner voice.

INVISIBLE FENCE

When I begged God to make me more like Christ, He gladly and seriously took me at my word. If you ask, it'll be the same for you. After God has taken you through circumstances that test you and reveal the sinfulness yet present in your heart, He will begin to prune you. At times you may feel as if you've gone from the pan of struggle directly into the fire of greater adversity. But God is simply cultivating you so that you may reflect His glory even more. John 15:8 teaches that the Lord desires that we bear much fruit to His Father's glory. So when there's a yielded branch abiding in the vine, God will indeed prune it so that it bears even more fruit.

In much the same way that a parent expects more and more from a child as he matures, God will also begin to expect more from you as you mature spiritually. For example, you'll eventually discover that things you once did—that you knew were displeasing to God yet felt not the slightest remorse about—you can no longer do, at least not without your conscience getting pricked. God has brought me to a place where now the mere thought of an intentional sin—that I could have done before and thought nothing of—unsettles my conscience. I also have a heightened awareness of when I fall short of God's glory, and now I more quickly seek His forgiveness and help. This multifaceted work of God in our hearts fortifies our spirit and empowers us to both resist temptation and walk away from sin.

The process whereby the Holy Spirit brings us into an awareness of sin is similar to an invisible fence. Before an invisible electrified fence is installed, a dog enjoys the carefree ability to go beyond the boundaries of his owner's property. He does so again and again and thinks nothing of it. After the invisible fence has been installed, the dog's training commences. Not long afterward, he begins to cautiously approach the familiar boundary that he previously would have gone beyond. Over time, he progressively learns to associate the shock he receives with having gotten too close to the newly established boundary. His carefree romps in the yard become curtailed as he gradually learns to steer clear of the invisible fence. Eventually, the dog loses his desire to go anywhere near the fence. And if the dog were to inadvertently wander too close to the fence, he would immediately sense the danger in going any farther—and he wouldn't want to. Instead, he'd turn around and quickly distance himself from the fence.

Because of our old, familiar fallen natures, we instinctively seek to gratify our flesh. Without the Holy Spirit's conviction, we will continually seek to satisfy our natural urges and desires—to go outside of God's boundaries for our lives, much like a dog wants to wander beyond its boundaries. Over time, we may even gain complete victory over the desire to commit the sins that once gratified our flesh, much like the dog loses his desire to go anywhere near the invisible fence.

EMBRACING THE CROSS

One of the primary reasons God allows us to walk through trials and struggles is so that we may see our desperate need of Him. He also shatters our satisfaction and preoccupation with temporal things so that we may learn to cleave to Him more.

Elisabeth Elliott captures this idea saliently:

God has allowed in the lives of each of us some sort of loss, the withdrawal of something we valued, in order that we may learn to offer ourselves a little more willingly, to allow the touch of death on one more thing we have clutched so tightly, and thus know fullness and freedom and joy that much sooner. We're not naturally inclined to love God and seek His kingdom. Trouble may help to incline us—that is, it may tip us over, put some pressure on us, lean us in the right direction. If through losing what this world prizes we are enabled to gain what it despises—treasure in Heaven, invisible and incorruptible— isn't it worth any kind of suffering? What is it worth to us to learn a little bit more of what the Cross means—life out of death, the transformation of earth's losses and heartbreaks and tragedies?[39]

....

39. Elisabeth Elliot, *Keep a Quiet Heart* (Grand Rapids: Revell, 2008), 39.

CHAPTER 16
SPIRITUAL WORKOUTS

> I know of no other way to triumph over
> sin long-term than to gain a distaste for it
> because of a superior satisfaction in God.
> —John Piper

Besides making us more like Christ, becoming filled with more of God also promotes wholehearted devotion. True devotion to God is a constant and determined desire to do what we know is pleasing to Him. The Bible teaches, "Run from anything that stimulates youthful lusts. Instead, pursue righteous living, faithfulness, love, and peace" (2 Timothy 2:22, New Living Translation). The goal of this chapter, therefore, is to provide practical information on how we can grow in our surrender to Christ by learning to resist temptation and to flee from sin (see James 4:7).

Our finite minds, coupled with the deceptive nature of sin, make it impossible for us to search our own hearts; we don't simply discover sin in our hearts—God must reveal it to us. Psalm 139:23–24 promises that if we humble ourselves before God and ask Him to search our hearts and minds, He will. As I've mentioned, God searches our hearts with the divine floodlight of His Word but, thankfully, never without it being plugged into the generator of His grace. God never reveals our sin to guilt, shame, or condemn us: "There is therefore now no condemnation for those who are in Christ Jesus" (Romans 8:1). God shows us our sins because He desires to set us free from things that have kept us in bondage. Therefore, any revelation that God gives will *always* be a gift of His tender mercies to deepen our understanding of our desperate need of His grace and to refine and mature us so that we progressively imitate Him.

God also lovingly shows us where we're missing the mark because gratifying our fleshly nature is contrary to His desire for us. God wants us to be released from sin's bondage in greater and greater degrees so that we may lead holy lives and increasingly experience the abundant life that our Savior died for us to have, including joy, hope, peace, confidence, boldness, and contentment. God also desires us to progressively experience the joy and freedom that come from a vibrant, intimate relationship with Him. Above all else, He desires to be magnified in us.

MAKING GOD A PRIORITY

I know from experience that a passionate relationship with God is elusive. Part of the reason for this is that our love for God is often based on who we've conjured Him to be rather than who He really is. As a result, we don't really know God—we have not truly tasted His goodness or feasted on the delights of His love. So amid all the distractions of life, coupled with our own self-absorption, it's very easy to have a back-burner love for God. Often, we tend to have more passion, energy, and enthusiasm for worldly pursuits, which eventually usurp God's place in our lives. God knows this proclivity of our hearts. Therefore, He lovingly commands us to not love the things of this world; to not be conformed to this world; to say no to ungodliness and worldly passions while saying yes to godly, self-controlled lives; and to avoid evil but cling to that which is good (see 1 John 2:15; Romans 12:2; Titus 2:12; Romans 12:9).

Something else steadily pushes God to the back burner of our lives: because of sin, we prefer to gratify ourselves more than we desire to please God. Pursuing our own goals slowly chips away at the desire to cultivate relationship with God. Eventually, we may completely brush God aside or just keep Him at the periphery of our lives. Either way, we end up justifying doing as we please.

For many of us, it's not that we don't love God or don't want to cultivate our relationship with Him. We really do; it's just that we can't seem to. We identify with Paul, who confessed that though in his inner being he delighted in God's law, it wasn't always demonstrated in his actions (see Romans 7:22). Paul states, "For I do not understand my own actions. For I do not do what I want, but I do the very thing I hate" (Romans 7:15). Even though he knew what was right to do, his fleshly passions kept getting in the way. He fervently yearned to love and obey God, yet still found himself falling short of God's desires.

Paul keenly realized that it was only through Christ's finished work on the cross that he could be delivered from his body of death (see Romans 7:25). All God's children share in this same blessed hope. It is only by faith that we can daily crucify the sinful deeds of the body and triumph over the schemes of Satan. He lures and entices us with what I call bitter candy: the bait of sin looks attractive and deliciously sweet, yet it is filled with spiritual poison that results in leanness of soul; all it takes is one bite to have the carnal or fleshly nature greedily wanting more. The more one eats of this bitter candy, the more one hungers after it.

NEVER SATISFIED

In the remainder of this chapter, we'll explore the process whereby we overcome temptation and put to death sin in our lives so that we increasingly delight God's heart. But first, we must understand how sin comes to gain greater and greater influence in our lives. We weaken our spiritual constitution each and every time we choose to deliberately sin. In so doing, we thicken the chains that keep us in bondage. Scripture says, "That which is born of the flesh is flesh, and that which is born of the Spirit is spirit" (John 3:6). Although this verse refers more directly to being "born again," it's also applicable to the gratification of sinful desires. Carnal flesh can only birth more carnal flesh. The more we indulge our fleshly desires, the more power these desires wield over us.

It's also a vicious circle, because the flesh is like a spoiled brat. It vehemently demands to get its way—it wants what it wants, when it wants it, and as long as it wants it. This is why sin so readily enslaves us. Because we want to satisfy sinful desires, we're easily tempted by whatever is dangled before the eyes of our heart. Before we even realize it, we've figuratively grabbed hold of the sin with both hands, much like Eve may have literally done with the forbidden fruit in the Garden.

The more we give in to our flesh, the more we lack the power to not give in to what it wants at a later time. As much as we may overlook this reality, choosing to give in to our flesh makes us weaker and weaker in our ability to say no to sinful desires. Over time, these sinful desires become stronger and sin more deeply entrenched. Left unchecked, our flesh will continually feed off our weakness to refuse its wishes. As a matter of fact, it increasingly makes stronger and stronger demands. For this reason, a person who constantly indulges his fleshly nature will naturally commit more sins than someone who intentionally restrains his desires. As the flesh gets more and more of its way, our consciences become callous or desensitized. We become more and more apathetic about the ramifications of sin, which often leads to even more serious sin—and our bondage becomes greater.

For example, here's a situation that often occurs, albeit to varying degrees, and it ties into the whole idea of sinking thinking discussed in Chapter 13. Someone is found guilty of embezzling $10,000 of company money. In all likelihood, this would not have been the person's first occasion to steal. He may have gotten his start in seemingly innocuous wrongs, such as using company property for personal use—using the company printer to make personal copies or taking petty office supplies home. This may then have escalated to cheating on his gas mileage expense report or misrepresenting how much company money was actually spent on a business lunch, which in turn may have expanded into misappropriation of small sums of money. By repeatedly doing any of these things, he would have continually weakened his ability to say no to successive temptations that confronted him. By the time he was tempted to misappropriate the $10,000, he had become enslaved to taking property that didn't belong to him and, therefore, unable to discipline himself to refrain.

ENTHRONING CHRIST IN OUR HEARTS

I call flesh that has been fattened as a result of frequently getting its way "happy flesh." When our flesh is continually happy, we are simply living to please ourselves. Even worse, God is dishonored as our self-seeking desires provide occasion for the enemy and his minions to not only use us as instruments of evil but also scoff at God.

As followers of Christ, we are called to magnify—not defame—His name. We exalt Christ as we enthrone Him in our hearts—as we depend on His indwelling presence to subdue fleshly desires. Therefore, we must embrace the truth that it is only by becoming slaves to Christ that we truly become free. As Charles Spurgeon said, "[if I] have Christ [as] the absolute monarch in my heart . . . [then] I want to give up all my liberty to Him, because I feel that I will never be free until I abdicate the Throne to Him, and that I will never have my will truly free until it is bound in the golden fetters of His sweet love."[40]

---

40. Charles Spurgeon, *The Fullness of Joy* (New Kensington: Whitaker House, 1997), 26.

Indeed, there's absolutely no other way to walk out the freedom that Christ died for us to have. I've learned firsthand that sitting on the throne of my heart makes me significantly more vulnerable to Satan's attacks and all the more enslaved to sin with its destructive and often far-reaching repercussions. For example, when I cared more about pleasing myself, my husband and I experienced significantly more disagreements. Each time that we did, I predisposed myself to becoming angry, which does not bring forth the righteousness that is pleasing to God (see James 1:20). My discontentment would sometimes last for a couple of days, greatly affecting both my overall mood and behavior. Of course, this sour attitude also trickled into my interactions with the children with whom God has blessed us. Inadvertently taking out my frustration on them, I would at times be short or lose my temper. Most importantly, living with a grudge hindered my fellowship with God. I'm so thankful that by God's grace, my husband and I rarely have such disagreements now, and even when we do, we quickly resolve them and move forward in peace and love.

As I look back on my spiritual growth, I realize that I had to put my flesh on a serious diet in order to decrease the amount of time I spent sitting on the throne of my heart. With God's help, I was progressively empowered to deny my flesh what it wanted. For example, there were times when rather than engaging in a negative discussion with someone who seemed to always ruffle my feathers, I learned to keep quiet and walk away. Or instead of grumbling or complaining aloud when one of the children didn't do what I had expected, I became better at saying a prayer for help instead. I can attest from experience that the flesh becomes less demanding and less controlling only as it is deprived of its desires. Therefore, the only antidote for subduing fleshly desires is to make our flesh leaner and leaner by not giving in to its demands. To be controlled less and less by one's flesh is to be led more and more by the Spirit of God. It is to become softer and more pliable in our Father's hands so that He can mold us after His heart—this voluntary yielding pleases Him.

This spiritual reality reminds me of an interesting story about dog-fighting I once heard (although I'm definitely not in favor of the sport). A man owned several fight dogs. He regularly had two of his dogs fight one another—and he could predict with 100 percent accuracy which of his dogs would win a given fight. One day a spectator asked, "How is it that you always know which dog will win?" The man replied, "That's easy! The one that I feed before the fight." So it is with the fight between our flesh and our spirit. In the daily battle with sin, the one we feed the most is without a doubt the one that wins.

BUILDING SPIRITUAL MUSCLE

Here's the amazing flip side to this spiritual dynamic: just as flesh gives birth to more flesh, so does spirit give birth to more spirit. As we cooperate with the Holy Spirit to not gratify our flesh, something begins to happen. We begin to feed our spirit instead. As we study, apply what we've learned from Scripture, pray, and depend on the Lord, spirit gives birth to more spirit. Therefore, whenever God gives us the grace to say no to our flesh, we are simultaneously saying yes to our spirit. We are actually building up our spirit. The more we build up our spirit, the more we are strengthened to say no to temptations and fleshly desires.

Before going on, I must mention that when we say no to sinful desires or habits, we will at first experience a kind of void. We must immediately fill that void with something good or godly as taught in both Matthew 12:45 and Luke 11:26. For example, if a person engages in a certain kind of sin, but then chooses to stop, he or she would need to fill that void with something else that is Christ-honoring. We see a similar dynamic when we fast: we willingly create a physical void in our lives by abstaining from food, TV, Facebook, sports, and then replace that emptiness with more of the Lord.

Here's an illustration of how we begin to build spiritual muscle: If a person wants to bench-press three hundred pounds, does he begin by making an immediate attempt to lift three hundred pounds? Of course not! He would start by first lifting a smaller weight, perhaps one hundred pounds, and then progress to heavier and heavier weights. Well, the process for putting to death our sinful desires is similar. We begin building spiritual muscle by refusing to gratify a carnal desire that we are actually able to lift—that is, a desire that we can already resist giving in to.

As an experiment, let's assign a particular fleshly desire a weight of five pounds. By repeatedly lifting it, we build spiritual muscle. Over time we discover that lifting that five pounds—aka denying that desire—is no longer as hard as it initially was. The very longing that was once hard to resist has now lost its power. We would have succeeded in making our flesh a little leaner while our spirit became a little stronger. We're on the right track, appropriating God's grace to walk out a more godly life that accords with our identity in Christ. This encourages us and fortifies our resolve to keep building spiritual muscle.

Now imagine being confronted with a ten-pound carnal desire, one that is quite a bit harder for us to lift or resist. However, as a result of our previous spiritual weight lifting, this new, heavier temptation— that would have otherwise gotten the best of us—is easier to deny, because we are spiritually stronger. Had we not built up our spiritual muscle by lifting or denying the five-pound desire, we might not have been able to deny this ten-pound desire.

So here's an important truth: barring a miraculous intervention (like when God delivers someone from an addiction and completely takes the desire away), we will likely never be able to deny a thirty-pound carnal desire if we have not first trained ourselves by saying no to less heavy carnal desires, any more than an average person can just walk off the street into a gym and bench-press three hundred pounds without any prior training. It just doesn't happen!

In the earlier example of embezzlement, we may think of the person who embezzled funds as giving in to a fifty-pound desire. Had he denied the five-pound desires to not have misused company property or chosen not to have fudged his mileage expense report, perhaps he would have built up enough spiritual fortitude to have resisted the fifty-pound temptation to embezzle the $10,000 when it presented itself.

The Bible warns us to resist temptation and flee from sin—running as far away as we can. Lingering near or courting temptation is like placing hay next to a roaring fire; it will surely be consumed.

THINK LEAN!

As you can see, thinking lean is not applicable to just our diet or physical health; it's very applicable to our spiritual health as well. Spiritual workouts—starting small and working our way up—pay great dividends. Every choice we make to sin—no matter how small—diminishes our ability to experience God in the moment. This is not to say that we can ever damage our relationship with God once we are His. I'm saying that the more we desire unbroken fellowship with God, the more we desire to deny the temptations we face, and the leaner our flesh becomes. I can't speak for you, but I never want to fall back into the same sins that God has given me the grace to overcome. Just like after modifying my eating habits and losing twenty pounds several years ago, I never want to go back to my previous weight.

Going lean is of great importance to God. As we continue to build spiritual muscle, our lives honor and glorify Him all the more. Training ourselves to deny our fleshly nature—by enriching our spirit—is ultimately birthed from the desire to be pleasing to God, a longing rooted in our recognition of God as the supreme end of our affections. Though we may fail miserably, we want to do all things for the glory of the one our hearts love. His delight and pleasure become both the motivation and the reward for all we do.

PRINCIPLE 5

VALUE AN ETERNAL MIND-SET

CHAPTER 17

FINDING OUR DELIGHT IN GOD

The worth and excellency of a soul is to be
measured by the object of its love.
—Henry Scougal

We've come to the last section of this book, where the rubber meets
the road—where we must view all of what we've so far learned as
having laid a foundation for us to press even deeper into God. Now
is a good time to honestly assess your relationship with God. Are you
overwhelmed by His amazing, unending love and as a result truly
delighting in Him? If not, do you at least have the desire to do so? I've
discovered that even if we're not where we want to be in our spiritual
journey, if we earnestly desire to want to make progress, we will. In
this chapter, we'll look at the primary obstacle that hinders us from
delighting in God. It's easily the grandest attraction that entices us to
override the directives of the divine GPS. Although the divine GPS
makes repeated attempts to redirect us, we're too smitten to notice its
recalibrations. Ignoring its guidance hinders our spiritual growth and
distances us from God. As we know, both outcomes greatly undermine
our ability to live backward.

ALLURITIS

We live in a world that is filled with lies and deception. According to John 8:44, this is due in large part to the fact that, Satan, the enemy of God's people, is a liar and the father of lies. His lies tempt us to chase after the glittering allurements and fleeting pleasures of this world, which all possess great power to ensnare us. All too easily, they take our focus away from God, competing for the devotion and allegiance He alone deserves. In so doing, they distract us from our central purpose to live for God's renown. I know what this is like because I used to be enticed to find satisfaction in the transient things of this world rather than in a vibrant relationship with God. If we don't recognize these empty things for what they really are, we'll inevitably chase after them in search of meaning or significance. The pursuit of them effectively blinds us, turning us astray from God's path for our lives.

Looking around, it seems many "Christians" have blindly walked into the traps of worldly enticements ever strewn on their paths. Having stumbled and fallen, they've sustained what I call alluritis, a spiritual concussion resulting from a preoccupation with worldly pleasures and the trappings of success. But the good news is that we serve the Greatest Physician. He has the power both to lead us away from the allurements that steer toward a spiritual concussion as well as to offer us the treatment to remedy it. So I want to throw light upon this malady to illuminate its destructive influence in our lives so that we may wholly set our hearts on loving God and living for His glory.

To one degree or another, virtually all of us have been infected by this soul-destroying ailment. Naturally, the severity of this acute spiritual condition may be assessed by the extent to which a person is chasing after wealth, success, security, happiness, and personal comfort to find significance in life. The most severe case occurs when the pursuit of temporal pleasures has become someone's sole focus in life.

Essentially, Christians with alluritis have lost sight of the truth that not only is God alone the source of true joy and contentment, He desires to be the object of our first love. Those with this spiritual heart disease haven't yet grasped that when we buy the hollow merchandise of this world, we stand in contempt of God's design—we emulate the self-seeking actions that the Israelites exhibited long ago. God's response to His people's turning away from Him conveys deep agony and longing, "for my people have committed two evils: they have forsaken me, the fountain of living waters, and hewed out cisterns for themselves, *broken* cisterns that can hold no water" (Jeremiah 2:13; emphasis mine). The things of this world hold out empty promises, because we find true and lasting fulfillment in none other than God. So besides forfeiting the joy, peace, victory, and contentment that come from an intimate relationship with God, those with this spiritual condition end up living as though the things amassed in this brief life are really what matter. God's Word makes it amply clear that "one's life does not consist in the abundance of his possessions" (Luke 12:15). God knows these things can never truly satisfy us.

DRIVEN BY PLEASURE

There's nothing inherently wrong with desiring pleasure. Actually it's been hardwired into us. It's a psychological fact that all mammals have an inherent desire to pursue pleasure and avoid pain. Therefore, whether or not we realize it, each of us avidly pursues some goal or activity simply for the sake of pleasure. Some desires are misguided. For example, some people are overly focused on themselves and derive great satisfaction from constantly seeking to make themselves fitter, stronger, or more beautiful. Other pleasures have potentially detrimental consequences, such as gambling away money that should have been used for essentials. Of course, some desires are perfectly fine, like someone who preoccupies herself with giving meaningful assistance to others.

The ultimate reason that God has given us this primal desire is so that we might seek and find pleasure in Him—in His beautiful and all-satisfying love. God created rocks, trees, animals, mountains, clouds, lakes, and a host of other animate and inanimate entities. They all exist to declare His glory. However, God does not desire to have a personal or loving relationship with these things. The fundamental reason we are made in God's image is so that, by possessing a measure of His likeness, qualities, and nature, we may enjoy fellowship with Him and Him with us.

In fact, part of Westminster Shorter Catechism of 1647 reads, "Man's chief end is to glorify God and enjoy Him forever." "In [God's] presence there is fullness of joy; at [His] right hand are pleasures for-evermore" (Psalm 16:11). It stands to reason that we can't enjoy God unless we first have a relationship with Him, much like a human being cannot enjoy intimacy with another human being outside of a close relationship with that person. This truth points right back to the importance of cultivating a passionate love relationship with God. We simply cannot glorify God with our lives if we aren't enjoying His fellowship and presence. In the same vein, we also cannot truly worship and adore a God whom we do not know and trust.

God desires to be uppermost in our affections—to be our first love (see Exodus 20:5, 34:14). It's His design that we have a passionate, intimate relationship with Him above all else. Therefore, He will *never* allow us to find true fulfillment or lasting contentment in anything or anyone apart from a vital, committed relationship with Himself. So many of us, I find, seem to be plain oblivious to this most critical reality. Here's a vital truth: we cannot build lives of true significance until we embrace that we were created for nothing less than a vibrant love relationship with our Creator—the God of the universe.

Referring to God, Revelations 4:11 declares, "You created all things, and by your will they existed and were created." That includes us. Integral to pleasing God is finding our greatest pleasure in Him. This truth is at the heart of God's declaration, "I am the Lord your God . . . You shall have no other gods before me" (Exodus 20:2–3). The Bible clearly teaches that God desires us to worship and adore Him alone: "You shall worship the Lord your God and him only shall you serve" (Matthew 4:10; see also Luke 4:8). However, we read this command and are tempted to think that God desires us to worship Him only for His benefit—that He made this decree because He is God. In so doing, we overlook the exciting truth that in giving us this sweeping command, He also has *our* pleasure and ultimate fulfillment in mind. God, who is omniscient, knows that our self-centered preoccupations and substitutions for Him can never satisfy the deepest longings of our souls; He alone can truly satisfy our deepest thirst and hunger because He alone is all-sufficient and all-satisfying.

WE ALL WORSHIP SOMETHING

Yet because of sin, we instinctively seek pleasure in everything but God. If we're not intentional, we will never earnestly seek fulfillment in God. And if we're not careful, the things that we pursue for pleasure— even the good things—will end up becoming idols in our lives. We may not bow down to these idols, but in a very real sense, we worship them. For example, some people worship themselves. Others worship their children, their favorite sports team, their career, their boat, their car, their beautiful lawn, an innate ability, or a specific passion. Still others worship false "religious" gods. Regardless of who we are or what we do, each of us worships something or some entity.

Because sin blinds us, many of us scarcely recognize the idols in our lives; if we do, we often don't view them as seriously as we ought or we rationalize and justify why we have them. Granted, not all idols have the same degree of weightiness; some are far worse than others. For example, there's a qualitative difference between a woman being preoccupied with having a tidy home but still making time for God versus a woman who actually worships her home, spending tremendous amounts of time, money, and energy in making it her castle to the exclusion of God.

We also fail to recognize that because our greatest joy should be found in our relationship with God, anything else from which we derive our greatest fulfillment is not only an idol, it also becomes our god. *It has taken the place of God in our lives!* Whether or not we realize it, when our primary joy is found in something or someone other than God, we violate the first and most fundamental commandment: to have no other gods besides God. This idolatry grievously dishonors God. In essence, our actions convey that whatever we worship or idolize is more desirable, more admirable, or more worthy of our time and affection than God Himself, who is the ultimate expression of love. To view something that God or man has created as having more intrinsic worth and value than God Himself is a woeful affront to God, for it calls into question His very perfections. Although we may not want to acknowledge it, having alluritis is practicing idolatry, because the pursuit of worldly goals or pleasures has actually become one's god.

THINK TWICE ABOUT FAME

The desire for personal fame, a rapidly growing preoccupation, is one manifestation of alluritis. To desire fame for the sake of personal ambition, recognition, significance, popularity, and the like is self-centered, not God-centered. It is to pursue one's own glory rather than God's glory. In a sense, it's a desire to worship oneself—one's success, talents, and achievements—rather than to worship and delight in the God who has actually bestowed these unmerited gifts. It's also a misdirected desire for others to make much ado about the creature (or person) at the expense of not glorifying the Creator.

As a matter of fact, a recent survey by the Barna Group "indicated that perhaps the most dangerous means to public awareness is through moral compromise."[41] This does not exclude Christians. As a whole, we continue to greatly compromise on biblical standards, increasingly conforming our lives to the secular values and patterns of this world. In addition, "recent studies have indicated that one of the most common goals among young Americans is to become famous. The wild popularity of reality TV shows and blogging are outgrowths of that urge."[42] Yet few would deny that the praise of this world is generally short-lived and often accompanied by much sorrow.

This pervasive desire for personal fame is Satan's distortion of our God-given desire to matter for His glory. It results in destructive tendencies, misconceived ideologies, and other preoccupations that literally destroy lives. An unhealthy desire for fame also ruins friendships, careers, and, most importantly, marriages and families.

If we need proof that fame or the quest for fame wrecks and destroys lives, we need look no further than Hollywood celebrity figures and their marriages. Their extremely high divorce rate relative to the mass population testifies that notoriety is not all it's cracked up to be. Although these celebrities have attained fame and recognition, having often reached the pinnacle of success in their given fields, news stories of their dissatisfied or wasted lives abound. Many are empty, miserably unhappy, and disillusioned with life. As a result, not only is suicidal depression prevalent, many celebrities have taken their own lives or made poor choices resulting in the loss of life.

....

41. "Billy Graham Tops Religious Leaders," Barna Group, accessed October 10, 2012, http://www.barna.org/barna-update/article/17-leadership/109-billy-graham-tops-religious-leaders?q=positive+views+christians.

42. Ibid.

BE CAREFUL WHAT YOU LOVE

In the end, the idols that we perceive as good and worthy of our time and energies end up literally destroying our lives and our souls. Truly, the world cannot satisfy us. It will always leave us empty, thirsty, and hungry.

Because of the pitfalls and destructiveness of idols that compete for God's place in our hearts, the Bible warns us to avoid the things of this world. Paul's stern words to the Corinthian church are just as applicable to the universal church today: "I beg of you that when I am present I may not have to show boldness with such confidence as I count on showing against some who suspect us of walking according to the flesh" (2 Corinthians 10:2). This Scripture is one of many which clearly teaches that, in order to please God, we must not walk after the flesh—patterning our lives after the secular values and misguided standards of this world. Rather, we are called to find our delight in God. This entails being completely out of step with the world's parade. We must also have our musical instruments tuned to a different pitch (see John 17:4). The resultant notes and melodies will then be out of harmony, creating music that is distinctly different than that of the world—music that honors God and pleases His heart. As we've seen, this is the singular pathway to our greatest delight and contentment.

Scripture also exhorts, "Do not love the world or the things in the world. If anyone loves the world, the love of the Father is not in him. For all that is in the world—the desires of the flesh and the desires of the eyes and pride of life—is not from the Father but is from the world. And the world is passing away along with its desires, but whoever does the will of God abides forever" (1 John 2:15–17). Misguided desires for pleasure, material possessions, and power cover each and every idol that we could metaphorically carve for ourselves.

If we truly love God and desire to delight in Him, we must be intentional about seeking His help to root out the sinful desires lurking in our hearts. Besides seducing us to pursue worldly things, these desires entice and tempt us, lure and bedazzle us, ensnare and entrap us, eventually bringing about our destruction.

It is in full view of these sinful desires and pernicious enemies to our soul that James issues this firm rebuke: "You adulterous people! Do you not know that friendship with the world is enmity with God? Therefore whoever wishes to be a friend of the world makes himself an enemy of God" (James 4:4). Like spiritual gasoline, this verse sets ablaze the fear of God in me. To consort with the world—regardless of the degree of our attachment—is to literally position oneself as an enemy of God. It is disheartening that many people who call themselves Christians actually live as enemies of God. They mindlessly believe that their adulterous lifestyles have God's smiling approval when, in reality, they are perilously living under His frowning countenance.

Exodus 34:14 states, "for you shall worship no other god, for the Lord, whose name is Jealous, is a jealous God." God is a jealous God, but not in the same sense that we use "jealous." We use this word to express our feeling when we wish we had something that someone else has. That God is jealous simply means that God will not tolerate one of His creations worshiping anything other than Himself. He will not share His glory with another. If you are His child, Jesus Christ is your beloved Bridegroom and you are a part of His bride. Jesus died to have a beautiful bride, without spot and wrinkle, and increasingly holy and devoted to Him (see Ephesians 5:27). The Bible plainly teaches that we have a love affair with the world when we frolic with worldly pleasures, giving the preponderance of our time, attention, devotion, and resources to them rather than to God. So to set one's affections on the things of this world is nothing less than spiritual adultery. It is to be unfaithful to Christ who displayed the greatest measure of love and unwavering commitment by suffering a most horrific death so that we may truly live.

Committing spiritual adultery, like adultery in a marriage, is not a pretty picture. God's heart is deeply grieved by the collective unfaithfulness of His children.

LEARNING FROM HISTORY

We can gain a better understanding of just how much our spiritual infidelity wounds the heart of God by looking at the self-serving actions of God's chosen people. The Old Testament depicts God's covenant with Israel as a marriage. On numerous occasions, Israel is portrayed as God's bride or wife who forsakes Him for other lovers. The depictions of Israel's spiritual adultery are very graphic and colorful, even repulsive at times. For example, Jeremiah 3:1 states, "'You have played the whore with many lovers; and would you return to me?' declares the Lord." Isaiah 57:8 adds, "Deserting me, you have uncovered your bed, you have gone up to it, you have made it wide; and you have made a covenant for yourself with them, you have loved their bed." And finally, Ezekiel 16:32 describes Israel as an "Adulterous wife, who receives strangers instead of her husband!"

I can think of nothing more lewd and blasphemous in all of God's Word. In fact, few verses of the Scriptures more deeply express God's intense grief and sorrow than the portrayals of Israel's prostitution and unfaithfulness. Their infidelity profaned a God infinitely deserving of praise, reverence, and adoration from the objects of His affection: His people. God's people repeatedly broke His heart and forsook His love despite all the miraculous and marvelous things He had done on their behalf. Israel's illicit love affairs with the pagan world around them aroused feelings of anger and unrequited love in God similar to those of someone whose spouse has been unfaithful.

These portrayals of Israel are painful reminders of God's jealous affection for His children. Just as a husband and wife desire wholehearted devotion from one another, so does God want our whole heart, not half of it, or any fraction, for that matter. In light of God's extrava-gant love for us, our idolatry and spiritual adultery seem to be the sins that He hates the most, as they offend Him—as well as His grace and mercy—the most.

These poignant depictions of Israel's adulterous affairs help guard my heart against the allure of this world and fortify my desire to never forsake my first love. If we, the bride of Christ, are devoted to and truly love God, Israel's lewd and sickening spiritual adultery should strengthen our resolve to keep our hearts undefiled by the world; it should instill a holy and righteous fear against ever wounding God's heart and spurning His love. To make progress in this area, we must be intentional about living in such a way that we continually uphold the truth that God is wholly desirable and worthy of our affection and devotion.

We must live more like the early Christians. Early Christians understood the grave need to separate themselves from the things of this world. They sold their goods and possessions and distributed them among themselves according to individual needs (see Acts 2:44–45, 4:32–35). Besides displaying a wonderful spirit of generosity, these gracious and selfless acts were proof positive that they were no longer attached to worldly goods. They were detached from the things of this world because they truly believed that they had found everything in Jesus. We can model their mind-set even if we don't sell all our posses-sions. At the same time, we must acknowledge that to look for satisfac-tion in the things of this world implies—especially *to the world*—that Jesus is not enough for us.

May we seek God's help to become increasingly disenchanted by the things of this world. May we pray that God would continually illu-mine us to the gods that we unknowingly love, serve, and adore. The gods that compete with the Lover of our Souls, creating huge barriers to a passionate relationship with Him. Then may we petition Him to give us the grace, wisdom, and fortitude of heart to decisively smash to pieces those idols that have usurped His rightful place in our hearts.

May we also pray that the door of our hearts would be barred shut when worldly desires come knocking, and that we would increasingly seek deeper and deeper intimacy with the one true King of our hearts. Ultimately, may we pray that our spiritual beds be kept undefiled, exclusively reserved for God and God alone. Then and only then can we affirm that He alone is our first love and supreme delight.

CHAPTER 18

....

THE PITFALLS OF MONEY AND POSSESSIONS

I find in the Bible a divine command to be a pleasure-seeker—
that is, to forsake the two-bit, low-yield, short-term, never-
satisfying, person-destroying, God-belittling pleasures of the
world and to sell everything in order to have the kingdom of
heaven and thus "enter into the joy of your master."
—John Piper

Forsaking the world to find our delight in God is most wonderful,
but we cannot stop there. To honor God and make the most of our
lives, it's also critical that we understand the self-destructive nature of
materialism. Only then can we stem its rapidly growing influence in
our lives.

THE BABY OF MATERIALISM

Materialism is a preoccupation with material rather than intellectual
or spiritual things. We live in a very materialistic culture where self-
absorption is the general way of life. A major outgrowth of this self-
absorption is that we are overly concerned about our status, especially

with respect to how we are perceived. Therefore, we might say that a preoccupation with our status is the baby of materialism. I've heard it said that status is "buying what you don't need with money that you don't have to impress others who don't care." This common behavior sounds pretty foolish when you think of it this way.

Picture the following things: a high-tech gadget that was purchased through an infomercial but has been used only once; a state-of-the-art bread maker that hasn't been used to make a single loaf of bread; a heart-rate monitor that has never once recorded a heart rate because it has never been worn; gardening magazines decorating a coffee table that have never been read.

In general, North Americans are obsessed with having the latest and greatest new technology, and the biggest and best appliances. We want others to see just how successful we are. This preoccupation with more, bigger, and better is like a terrible epidemic. I came across the following definitions for a term called affluenza:

1. The bloated, sluggish and unfulfilled feeling that results from efforts to keep up with the Joneses.

2. An epidemic of stress, overwork, waste and indebtedness caused by dogged pursuit of the American Dream.[43]

In fact, several years ago, PBS aired a television special called "Affluenza." It highlighted some startling facts in our "modern-day plague of materialism"[44]:

• A higher percentage of Americans have declared bankruptcy than have graduated from college.

• The average American spends a meager forty minutes a day interacting with his or her children while, by comparison, spending a whopping six hours a week shopping.

The show's producers aired the program to tell people that affluence simply does not make us happy. The show discussed overconsumption

43. "Affluenza," PBS, accessed December 4, 2012, http://www.pbs.org/kcts/affluenza/.
44. Ibid.

and put a spotlight on the reality that the pursuit of materialism does not satisfy us.

Furthermore, materialism is self-centered, because it makes a god of our desire for recognition (from others) based on our perceived status. Like all self-centered goals, it deceives us to take our focus off God and His purpose for our lives. Clearly, this beguiling distraction undermines our ability to live backward.

THE MISPLACED PRIORITIES OF PROSPERITY AND WEALTH

It is not inherently wrong to make or accumulate more money, provided that we don't idolize it or become ensnared by it. I want to emphasize that God has given some individuals both the grace and wisdom to handle wealth in ways that are indeed pleasing to Him (for example, being generous givers or willing to part with all accumulated money at God's request). However, in general, money has an unobtrusive way of owning us and yanking our hearts away from God, undermining our relationship with Him and hindering His plan for our lives. The peril of having lots of money is that there's an ever-present danger to entirely forget about God as we find ourselves slaves to the kinds of happiness it can buy.

The desire to increase one's material comforts and social capital is a subtle but deep-rooted idolatry. Like the desire for fame, materialism is a lie of the enemy that deceives us into elevating God's gifts over God Himself. It places an inordinate value on the fleeting things of this world, because it makes mere personal comfort and luxury the be-all and end-all in life. We greatly dishonor God when we look to the empty things of this world for meaning and significance. All in all, a preoccupation with worldly pursuits effectively blinds us to the true spiritual condition of our hearts. In the previous chapter, we saw in James 4:4 that friendship with the world is enmity toward God. This verse only alludes to the desire to amass wealth for selfish reasons. In 1 Timothy

6:9–10, however, this topic is addressed head-on: "But those who desire to be rich fall into temptation, into a snare, into many senseless and harmful desires that plunge people into ruin and destruction. For the love of money is a root of all kinds of evils. It is through this craving that some have wandered away from the faith and pierced themselves with many pangs."

Despite this clear truth, many followers of Christ are enamored with wealth, actively pursuing it for wholly or partially self-centered reasons. I used to be one of those people. As mentioned earlier, my desire for wealth was rooted in the mistaken belief that I could find a measure of significance by achieving a certain level of worldly success or prosperity. But chasing after money and possessions amounts to chasing after the wind. Proverbs 23:5 (New Living Translation) states, "In the blink of an eye wealth disappears, for it will sprout wings and fly away like an eagle." Moreover, the desire for financial prosperity knits our heartstrings more tightly to the transient things of this world. This is why Hebrews 13:5 instructs, "Keep your life free from love of money, and be content with what you have." We can apply this principle to the pursuit of status symbols and worldly success as well.

DIMINISHING RETURNS

To our great detriment, the pursuit of material gain follows the principle of diminishing returns. Having the very things that we desire or crave eventually leads to increasingly less satisfactory results. For instance, take overeating. The fuller we are, the less tasty the food becomes. More importantly, continued overindulgence has great potential to erode both our health and self-esteem. Similarly, someone motivated by greed might insist on working longer and longer hours, eventually wrecking his marriage and destroying his family. In both examples, the desire for more actually results in a greater loss.

Over time, the things that we covet sicken our hearts, corrupt our souls, and bankrupt our lives. Indeed, an ever-increasing desire for an ever-diminishing pleasure is nothing short of sheer folly. And because this reality goes largely unrecognized, we don't realize just how much it serves to attach us even more to the pleasures and enticements of this fallen world. Consequently, we increasingly live for the things of this world while progressively becoming more apathetic that these desires are contrary to God's will for our lives, which are but a vanishing mist. And we forget all about our future heavenly existence. Again and again, we lose sight of the truth that each and every choice we make in the here and now has eternally profound consequences.

Jesus taught a poignant lesson on the desire for wealth. Mark 10:17–27 relates the story of a rich man who wanted to follow Jesus. When Jesus told him of the costs, he was unwilling to do so as it meant parting with his money. In response to the man's shortsighted decision, Jesus told his disciples, "How difficult it will be for those who have wealth to enter the kingdom of God!" (Mark 23). Jesus was not jesting with his disciples. Indeed, it is hard for the rich to enter His kingdom. In fact, Scripture seems to suggest that having wealth is most likely a spiritual liability rather than a spiritual asset (see Mark 10:23–25).

This scriptural reality raises a most sobering question. If Jesus said that it is hard for the rich to enter His kingdom, then why do we desire the very thing that makes our entrance into it all the more difficult? If the greatest blessing we can receive from God is the privilege of being a part of His kingdom—including all the temporal blessings that it carries—then how can we not believe that the desire for wealth may leave us as spiritually disadvantaged as the rich man? Why do we mindlessly overlook that, besides being a major obstacle to our continued spiritual growth, a preoccupation with wealth can cause us to forfeit many of the spiritual riches God desires to bestow on us during our earthly journey? And why would we want to position ourselves to be at a greater risk of forfeiting not only temporal but eternal blessings as well?

Consider this. If God wanted to curse someone, it seems one of the easiest and most decisive ways is to make that person very, very rich. Viewing their prosperity as the result of their own abilities and efforts, they can easily fall into the dangerous trap of relying on their wealth instead of depending on God. This pitfall of money is plainly taught in 1 Timothy 6:17: "As for the rich in this present age, charge them not to be haughty, nor to set their hopes on the uncertainty of riches, but on God, who richly provides us with everything to enjoy."

CLASSIC CASE STUDY ON WEALTH

The book of Ecclesiastes throws much light on the dangerous effects of wealth. The truth that wealth (or the desire for wealth) often brings about spiritual devastation is epitomized in the life of Solomon, the richest man who ever lived. After many futile attempts to find meaning in his wealth, including amassing gold and silver, building massive projects, and assembling a huge harem to fulfill his sexual desires, Solomon boasted, "Whatever my eyes desired I did not keep from them. I kept my heart from no pleasure, for my heart found pleasure in all my toil, and this was my reward for all my toil" (Ecclesiastes 2:10). He became puffed up by his power and influence. Over time, Solomon allowed his possessions to possess him.

The enticement of sinful desires and the progression of spiritual blindness compound on themselves. Solomon hopefully discovered the peril of sinful desires—they are ever-ready to court temptation. That is, we so easily succumb to temptations because they are so appealing to our sinful desires. If this were not true, temptations, in and of themselves, would lose much of their power to entice us.

As we've learned, the more we give in to temptations, the more we gratify sinful desires and, in turn, the more potent these desires become. This is why the more Solomon indulged his sinful passions, the more indulgent and reckless he became—to the point of eventually denying himself not a single pleasure. In the final analysis, Solomon was seduced and led astray by his own sinful desires—the lust of the flesh, the lust of the eyes, and the pride of life. And when his sin had given birth, it led to his spiritual ruin. After all the "greatness" that he had attained, all that Solomon could say was, "Then I considered all that my hands had done and the toil I had expended in doing it, and behold, all was vanity and a striving after wind, and there was nothing to be gained under the sun" (Ecclesiastes 2:11).

THE FUTILITY OF WEALTH

Solomon's fateful discovery is only accentuated by an interesting human tendency. Many who are hungry for fame, wealth, applause, prestige, and success are often limited by financial constraints. In the back of their minds, they hope that one more lucrative business deal, one more successful acting role, or one more promotion will finally make them feel fulfilled. Unrealized hopes and dreams spur them on.

By contrast, Solomon's great wealth, power, and abundant resources afforded him any desire of his heart. Like many wealthy folks today, there was nothing that he couldn't have or attain. Yet, also like those of today, despite all that he had at his disposal, Solomon was miserably empty and unfulfilled. Current statistics indicate that the extremes of both poverty and wealth are associated with higher suicide rates.[45] With regard to the latter, the high suicide rate among the rich may be intrinsically linked to the fact that a person becomes very disillusioned when he can have anything money and power can buy yet still finds happiness elusive. Empty and despairing, life loses meaning and all hope seems lost; people take their own lives because they believe their lives are no longer worth living.

....

45. Community Counseling Services, Inc., "Suicide Statistics," accessed May 15, 2015, http://www.hsccs.org/poc/view_doc.php?type=doc&id=13737.

As great as Solomon was, perhaps the only thing that exceeded his fame was the eventual futility of his life. The final chapters of his life story epitomize a wasted life. In the end, what good did Solomon's wealth afford him? Nothing but utter misery and despair, since "one's life does not consist in the abundance of his possessions" (Luke 12:15). Thousands of years later, many followers of Christ have not grasped this biblical lesson. Blinded by vain or self-driven ambition, we continue to think that money will once and for all give us the key to unlock the door in our hearts that leads to happiness and satisfaction. But it never can and never will.

LESSONS WE CAN LEARN

The Bible teaches, "For whatever was written in former days was written for our instruction, that through endurance and through the encouragement of the Scriptures we might have hope" (Romans 15:4). Here are several nuggets we can take away from the life of Solomon regarding materialism and the pursuit of wealth:

Materialism affords increased opportunities to fall into greater temptations and sins. The more we have, the more we want.

Materialism tempts us to find contentment in things of this world rather than in God. This false sense of security is one of the great deceptions of wealth. Few are humbled and spiritually grounded enough to view and handle wealth in ways that are pleasing to God.

Materialism leads to pride. We attribute our success to ourselves and progressively become less dependent on God as the true Source of all that we have. We're also tempted to become more ungrateful, which only increases our ability to become resistors, not conductors, of God's grace.

The pursuit of materialism blinds us to the simple joys of life, because having much in the way of material possessions typically means having that much more to manage, control, maintain, and worry about. This tyranny of possessions, similar to the tyranny of the routine, undermines our ability to invest in that which truly matters, such as time with family, time to study and meditate on God's Word, and giving of one's time to a worthy cause.

Materialism robs God of glory, because we passionately seek His gifts while we are dispassionate about Him; it robs us of the joy of being God's instrument to bless others; it robs others of our financial and material assistance; and, ultimately, it robs us of eternal treasures and rewards.

Materialism takes our focus off our ultimate purpose, which is to grow in Christlikeness. It also causes us to turn our focus away from feasting on the delights of worshiping and enjoying the all-sufficient God of the universe. As a result, we delight in our idols and self-centered desires.

We must learn to increasingly embrace the teaching of Matthew 6:24: "No one can serve two masters. Either you will hate the one and love the other, or you will be devoted to the one and despise the other. You cannot serve both God and money."

BUYING WHAT TRULY SATISFIES

Proverbs 11:4 instructs, "Riches do not profit in the day of wrath." The Bible clearly teaches that we each will have to account for our lives before God. On that fateful day, money will be utterly worthless. C. S. Lewis captured the idea of living unencumbered by the appeal of wealth or worldly goods: "He who has God and everything has no more than he who has God."[46] Truly, everything we could ever need is found in God.

One of my favorite verses in all of Scripture is Isaiah 55:1–2: "Come, everyone who thirsts, come to the waters; and he who has no money,

---

46. Cited in Randy Alcorn, *Money, Possessions, and Eternity* (Wheaton: Tyndale House Publishers, Inc., 2003), 3.

come, buy and eat! Come, buy wine and milk without money and without price. Why do you spend your money for that which is not bread, and your labor for that which does not satisfy? Listen diligently to me, and eat what is good, and delight yourselves in rich food."

There it is in black and white. The sweetest and single most precious thing in all the universe worth buying absolutely cannot be bought. Not with money, or anything else for that matter. Salvation, though it cost God everything, is free! And it is undeservedly ours. I've heard GRACE described as God's Riches At Christ's Expense. Because of this grace, God is our God and we are His people—forever and ever. Although it is a mind-boggling reality, our mortal lives will someday become immortal. Forever is never-ending! And the endless possibilities and opportunities God has in store for us should dull our materialistic desires and get us flat-out excited about living backward.

CHAPTER 19

·······························

BUILD A PORTFOLIO OF ETERNAL TREASURES

Whatever good thing you do for Him, if done according to the
Word, is laid up for you as treasure in chests and coffers, to be
brought out to be rewarded before both men and angels, to
your eternal comfort.

—John Bunyan

Besides developing godly character and wisely redeeming our
time on earth, no other activity carries greater weight than our
biblical stewardship of money. Taken together, these three spiritual
commodities make up the essential components of living backward.
In this chapter, we'll look at this third component: cultivating a God-
centered approach toward our use of money. We'll first dismantle our
false perspective on how we view money, and then we'll explore its
proper and biblical place in our lives.

NOT YOUR WILL BUT MINE BE DONE

Our use of money is perhaps the biggest area in our lives where
God's will and our desires go their separate ways. This reality hints

at why there are twice as many scriptural verses that relate to money (roughly two thousand) than to faith and prayer combined (about one thousand). In fact, more than 15 percent of everything Jesus taught was on the topic of money and possessions—which is also more than His teachings on Heaven and Hell combined. So why do we invariably find it hard to submit to God in the area of finances? Besides our stubbornness to submit to God due to sin, one of the most important factors is that we've been conditioned by the world's system to believe that the money we possess is actually ours to do with as we please.

Yet Scripture teaches that God owns everything: "The earth is the Lord's, and the fullness thereof" (Psalm 24:1). In reality, money and everything else that we're blessed to have has been entrusted to us by God. We are mere stewards—all that we have has always been and will always be God's. In the same way that a financial comptroller should have no challenge writing a business check in accordance with the CEO's request because the money isn't his, we should never be reluctant to part with any money that God has entrusted to us. I admit that this is a difficult teaching to embrace. After all, *we* want to decide how much money we give to a charity or to a special outreach collection at church. However, we can't simply ignore this key scriptural reality and go on treating God's money as though it is ours. Rather, we must live with open hands.

TRUTH AND CONSEQUENCES

Besides disobeying God, two things happen when we tightly hold on to His money and continue to do with it as we please. First, God will often withhold other, often better, gifts from us because our hands are figuratively closed. Second, we forfeit opportunities that carry eternal rewards to be channels of God's grace, through which He desires to bless both us and others.

It was a sobering moment when God showed me that I had made an idol of money, because I was unwilling to allocate it the way that He desired. Not only is money an idol for many of us, it has also come to replace God as the object of our trust. When we rely on our finite understanding to make financial decisions—big or small—and then allow those same decisions to supersede God's infinite wisdom and divine will, we have actually put our trust in money. By placing our confidence in man (in this case, ourselves) and "our" money, we contradict the biblical instruction: "It is better to take refuge in the Lord than to trust in man" (Psalm 118:8). I pleaded guilty on both counts back then, but I'm happy to add that over the years the Lord has helped me to develop a more God-centered view of money.

The Bible teaches that Satan is the prince of darkness or the prince of this world because He has contaminated the entire world with his sins (see John 14:30). He's also the lord of money. He is delighted when God's people are deceived about the potentially destructive power and harmful influence that money can wield in our lives. He's also thrilled when followers of Christ lack a biblical understanding of the proper place of money (and possessions). Satan wants us to go through life believing that how we view and use money is inconsequential and has no eternal bearing on our lives. However, nothing could be further from the truth. In fact, the consequences of making an idol of money are grave, precisely because they carry eternal ramifications. How we view and utilize money decisively determines what we truly value in this brief life; more sobering, it also influences the quality of the commendation that we receive in the eternal life to come.

Clearly, there's a great need for God's people to be grounded in a biblical understanding of money. We must grasp that how we utilize His money reveals a significant characteristic or heart index. That's because our willingness to part with God's money is an indicator of whether our hearts are attached to it. If we're genuinely unattached, then Jesus, not money, is enthroned on our hearts. It also means that we view money simply as a tool, not as an idol that we unknowingly serve.

As such, money emphatically reveals whether we are leveraging the gift of future-oriented hindsight and living backward. It determines whether we are living only for this vapor of life or living in light of eternity, whether we are truly devoted to God or in love with the hollow and transient things of this world.

STEWARD OR OWNER?

We must also recognize that how we use money in any given instance is never a neutral transaction. Each and every time that we spend money, we ultimately are furthering either God's kingdom or Satan's (which includes anything that gratifies our sinful or self-centered desires). Moreover, our use of money reveals whether we have bought into the heresy that we can do as we please with the money entrusted to us by God in this present life, yet not experience any grave negative consequences of our disobedience in the next. As I've stated, whatever money we have is not ours to do with as we please.

God cares a whole lot about how we spend *His* money. Perhaps the most fundamental reason that God cares so much is this: if Christ is not Lord over our money, then it follows that He is not Lord over every area of our lives. We can learn much about how God desires us to use money from two similar parables (see Matthew 25:14–30; Luke 19:11–27). They both relate to servants being held accountable for how they used the talents (monetary measures) entrusted to them by their master. The master's final commendation was based entirely on how each servant used the talents and funds assigned to him. So it will be with us someday. If Christ is indeed our Lord, we must heed the lessons in these parables. We cannot live our fleeting lives indifferent to our Master's numerous commands concerning money while mindlessly assuming that all will be well for us in eternity. Though salvation is unequivocally not at stake here, the quality of our eternal well-being is.

It goes a long way to think of our eternal well-being in terms of an eternal portfolio. There's a direct relationship between our attitude toward money now and the quality of our eternal condition. This principle may be illustrated by looking at how two biblical characters used the money that had been entrusted to them. The first account is found in Luke 12:18–19 where a wealthy man mused, "This is what I'll do. I will tear down my barns and build bigger ones, and there I will store my surplus grain. And I'll say to myself, 'You have plenty of grain laid up for many years. Take life easy; eat, drink and be merry.'"

By the looks of his accomplishments, this was indeed a very successful man—living the fullness of the good life, by today's standards. Yet God rebuked this wealthy man with these words, "'Fool! This night your soul is required of you, and the things you have prepared, whose will they be?' So is the one who lays up treasure for himself and is not rich toward God" (Luke 12:20–21).

We woefully delude ourselves if we don't realize that we risk incurring God's rebuke for attempting to amass worldly goods and seeking to live a comfortable life like the wealthy fool. The modern version of this twofold pursuit is akin to chasing after the American Dream—as we've seen, it's a materialistic pursuit driven by self-centered desires that doesn't advance God's kingdom.

It behooves us to pause and consider that Jesus told this wealthy man his priorities were out of order. He was a fool both for making plans as though his life were in his own hands and for hoarding "his" stuff. Here is John Piper's wise advice to anyone enamored of amassing the things of this world: "Quit being satisfied with the little 5 percent yields of pleasure that get eaten up by the moths of inflation and the rust of death. Invest in the blue-chip, high-yield, divinely insured security of Heaven. Devoting a life to material comforts and thrills is like throwing money down a rat hole."[47]

THE LEAST BECOMES THE MOST

Now let's contrast this wealthy man's view of money and material goods with the woman who Jesus put the spotlight on in another teaching. According to Mark 12:41–44, this poor widow put two copper coins into the temple treasury. This act was truly remarkable because the two coins represented all the money that she had. Jesus had been watching intently and was very impressed by what the widow had done. He promptly turned her sacrificial giving and generosity into a lesson for his disciples. Jesus told them, "Truly, I say to you, this poor widow has put in more than all those who are contributing to the offering box. For they all contributed out of their abundance, but she out of her poverty has put in everything she had, all she had to live on" (Mark 43–44).

We can only imagine how, in eternity, God will handsomely recompense this widow for her selfless giving. Over two thousand years later, God still desires his parable on giving to be a lesson for you and me to emulate as well.

Without the wisdom of Scripture, we'd mistakenly presume that the wealthy man was wise for skillfully and diligently employing his business acumen, whereas the widow was unwise or foolish for giving away the only bit of money that she had. This presumption underscores that our most basic beliefs and attitude toward money are generally contrary to God's. After all, Scripture clearly teaches that the wealthy man was *not wise*, and the poor widow was *not foolish*.

Invariably, history repeats itself. It's undeniable that many of God's children today have fallen prey to the same desires and ambitions displayed by the rich fool. We, too, desire to figuratively build bigger

---

47. John Piper, *Desiring God* (Sisters: Multnomah Books, 2003), 129.

barns. We have seemingly forgotten that, in addition to how we've used our gifts and time on earth, one day God will demand of us an account of how we have spent His money. It seems that many Christians are placing far too much emphasis on worldly things and, by comparison, far, far too little on their eternal futures.

This is in stark contrast to Jesus's teaching, "Do not lay up for yourselves treasures on earth, where moth and rust destroy and where thieves break in and steal, but lay up for yourselves treasures in Heaven, where neither moth nor rust destroys and where thieves do not break in and steal" (Matthew 6:19–20). In glossing over this principle, we're unwittingly impoverishing the overall quality of our eternal existence.

STEWARDSHIP 101: DETACHMENT REFLECTS SURRENDER

To heed our Master and be pleasing to God in the area of our finances, we must walk out biblical stewardship. It bears repeating that everything we are blessed with belongs to God and God alone; we own nothing—not even ourselves (see 1 Corinthians 6:19). Every tangible and intangible thing entrusted to us—money, spiritual gifts, talents, abilities, and worldly goods—can either be used as a tool to serve God's purposes or misappropriated to serve our self-centered goals. When a God-given talent or tool is not used for its intended purpose of glorifying God, it becomes an earthen trinket. By contrast, tools or talents that are used to honor God translate into eternal treasures.

Ask yourself: Am I patterning my life after Jesus's teachings on money, or have I allowed the desire for comfort and the pursuit of worldly stuff to dictate how I invest God's money? How we respond is an accurate gauge of whether we are storing up eternal treasures or forfeiting them. When we view money through the lens of an eternal perspective, we are motivated to purposefully invest it in treasures above. Conversely, a shortsighted view of money keeps us preoccupied with amassing treasures on earth. Due to sin, we all are naturally predisposed to this mistaken view. For this reason, we must be all the more vigilant with our choices concerning money.

In Chapter 13, we discussed how our thoughts are an index of our true spiritual condition. In a similar way, our degree of attachment to money is an accurate reflection of who we really are. If God will someday judge the life stories that we're building and the character that we're forging, then how we've handled His money is inextricably woven into each of our stories and our characters. Failing to have a biblical understanding of money undermines our growth in Christ and eternally affects our lives. We must bear in mind that while money affords us many of life's comforts and pleasures, it cannot buy a good reputation, godly character, or a right relationship with God—not now, and certainly not in eternity. If we're truly seeking to put God first, we will continually nurture the right perspective and attitude regarding both money and possessions. It's also important to recognize that the degree of our detachment from money—in the sense of how freely and willingly we put it at God's disposal—speaks volumes about the degree of our surrender to Christ as our Lord. As we grow in the fullness of Christ, we also grow in submission to His lordship. Similarly, as our understanding of biblical stewardship grows, so does the lordship of Christ in our lives: the more detached we are from money, the more surrendered we are and the more easily we place it at God's disposal. Of course, the opposite is true: the more attached we are to money, the less surrendered we are and the more difficulty we have putting it at God's disposal.

Since we are called to progressively become more like Christ, our attitude toward money should be characterized by an ever-growing surrender. We'll continue to dishonor God and fail in the area of biblical stewardship so long as we view the money entrusted to us as ours to do with as we please. However, as we become more surrendered, we'll increasingly view money as a tool to serve God's purposes and not our own. We'll gradually allow God to do as He pleases, not just with financial resources, but with everything else that He has entrusted to us.

THE FINANCIALLY FISCAL EMPLOYEE

How do we go about learning to earnestly view the money we handle as not belonging to us but to God? Imagine the CEO of the small company where you work enlisted your help to purchase a list of foods and supplies for an upcoming company picnic. Would you go to a wholesale food club like Costco or BJ's to buy the supplies and buy whatever *you* please while you're there? No! You'd know full well that the money to make the purchase is not yours, and you wouldn't be tempted to spend it on anything else—you'd stick to the list.

Moreover, the CEO has informed you that in keeping with company policy, the accounting department must have every expense verified with a receipt. So at every point in your shopping, you'd be fully aware that you're accountable to the company for each and every item purchased. You'd take this responsibility seriously, and you'd take the utmost precaution not to misplace or lose a single receipt. At all times you would be keenly aware that the money belonged to the company; likely, you wouldn't even consider using it for personal means.

What would happen if we started to think of God's money more in this way? Satan and the world have both deceived us into thinking that there's no one but ourselves to be accountable to. In general—barring expenses being shared with a spouse for budgetary purposes—there's no one demanding an account of how we've spent each dollar on any given day. As a result, our spending habits can go unchecked. We deceive ourselves in thinking there is no one to whom we're accountable, but just as Jesus watched what was being put into the temple treasury more than two thousand years ago, He's observing how we utilize the money God has entrusted to us today. We're accountable to Him for every penny of it.

Although we don't have to give an account for our spending today, the Bible tells us that God will one day summon us to give an account (see Jeremiah 17:10; Romans 14:12; 2 Corinthians 5:10). He will inquire as to how we used that which He entrusted to us for the advancement of His kingdom. What did we spend it on? Whom did we use it to help? Did we wisely invest it or did we squander it? Will we be able to give the Lord a good report? These questions are worthy of our serious evaluation.

The final question is the heart of the matter. No doubt, in eternity, each of us wants Christ to look at us and approvingly say, "Well done, good and faithful servant." I'd like to believe that is a large part of your motivation for reading this book. If we want to be commended as good and faithful servants *at that moment*, we must be good and faithful stewards *now*. Certainly, we won't be able to plead ignorance of Christ's teachings concerning money—God has given us His Word to instruct us in all things. As we've seen, several of Jesus's teachings and parables command us to be good stewards.

Good financial stewardship is not optional for true followers of Christ. It is not something that we can overlook if we really want to honor Christ with our lives. Indeed, it's a flagrant affront to God to have a greater fear of the temporal repercussions of mismanaging a company's money than we have of God's eternal judgments for mismanaging His.

WORKING FOR THE KINGDOM CFO

I encourage you to take a firm stand for Christ and to no longer buy into the false dictates of the world's system. As we engage this present life, may we earnestly endeavor to "stick to God's list." I pray that we each would begin to see ourselves as an employee of the kingdom, that we would exercise diligence and figuratively "save and show the receipts" to our kingdom CFO. Whether it's meeting a genuine need of ours or giving to a worthwhile cause, may we be wise stewards, carefully justifying the expenditures we make in light of both kingdom business and our eternal future. With each and every expense—no matter how little—may we ask ourselves: Does this directly or indirectly contribute to the robustness of God's kingdom's economy on earth?

We simply can't advance God's kingdom on earth so long as we're preoccupied with building our own. What might building our own kingdom look like? This will vary from one individual to the next, but, for me, it looked like periodically spending both time and money seeking out great deals to decorate the beautiful home I was blessed with. For someone else, it might be spending excessive amounts of money to maintain the most meticulous lawn in the neighborhood or to highlight one's home with an impressive landscape design. For many, it might be augmenting an already substantial wardrobe and shoe collection or spending money frivolously on personal amenities. For others, motivated by status or unconcerned about excess, it may be patronizing Starbucks every day instead of making coffee at home.

I'm not suggesting that we should never treat ourselves to a massage or indulge in a Starbucks Frappuccino from time to time. However, we often spend money carelessly without giving any thought to God's desires or the advancement of His kingdom, so let's be candid about what Scripture teaches. God has not called us to cater to our self-centered wants and desires when there's so much need among His people. Instead, we are called to invest God's money in ways that we know will not only be pleasing to Him but also will serve His purposes on the earth.

Cultivating this God-centered mind-set will radically alter our spending habits. It definitely has changed mine. For example, I avoid making flippant purchases when I call to mind that many of God's children throughout the world don't even have clean drinking water or basic food to eat. Continually redirecting my focus to these huge unmet needs strengthens my resolve to not be wasteful with the money God has entrusted to me. I'm also very mindful of the teaching: "Let each of you look not only to his own interests, but also to the interests of others" (Philippians 2:4). Truly, God has blessed us so that we might be a blessing to others.

We should also be challenged by the following teaching: "Tell [the rich] to use their money to do good. They should be rich in good works and generous to those in need, always being ready to share with others. By doing this they will be storing up their treasure as a good foundation for the future so that they may experience true life" (1 Timothy 6:18–19, New Living Translation). Relative to the poor of this world, if you own a house and a car, then you are one of "the rich" in this present world to whom Paul is referring in the above scripture.[48] We are those whom God has called to live selflessly and generously, showing good deeds toward the poor, homeless, broken, displaced, downtrodden, and disadvantaged.

KINGDOM-SHRINK

In Old Testament times, the temple in which God's people worshiped Him had three distinct areas. In order of distance from the Ark of the Covenant that represented God's presence with His people, there was the outer court, the inner court, and the holy of holies (where the ark was situated). This temple setup illustrates the biblical mandate to use the wealth God has entrusted to us for His purposes: this teaching must move from the outer court of our minds to the inner court of our hearts and then practically into our lives so that God is honored with what He has entrusted to us. This means taking to heart that a servant is not above His master. This particular teaching, by the way, is found in five separate passages: Matthew 10:24; Luke 6:40; John 13:16; John 15:20; and Acts 17:11. Jesus lived a simple life on earth. As His disciples, we are called to do the same. There's a big difference between a want and a need. God has promised to supply all our needs (see Philippians 4:19), not necessarily provide for our wants. God wants

----

48. "Am I Rich?," Remember the Poor, accessed May 14, 2015, http://iremberthepoor.org/3-2/.

us to be diligent about seeking out opportunities to be a blessing to others, thus bringing His name more renown.

I heard an insightful quote from the movie *Confessions of a Shopaholic*. The facilitator of the protagonist's shopaholic support group admonished her, "You're willing to give your money away for things that you don't need, so why not try giving away the things you don't need for no money?" Instead of buying more stuff that we don't really need or can't afford (to impress people who really care far less about what we have than we think), how about kingdom-shrinking— periodically take stock of what we no longer need and prayerfully ask God what we should do with those items.

Many of us, including myself, may at the same time have to repent and ask God's forgiveness for acquiring goods and services with His money that we never should have purchased in the first place. Things we simply wanted that likely didn't come close to qualifying as a genuine need. Then, as much as our flesh may scream and cry out in pain, we should give away those things we no longer require, honoring the poor and needy as God has instructed us to do. I personally need to get busier with this activity; a friend donates regularly and experiences the blessing of freedom from the tyranny of possessions.

Granted, Scripture teaches that there will always be those who lack material needs. However, we can choose today to be God's instruments to alleviate some of the inequities in the world. For those who do, God has given this rich promise: "There is one who is free in giving, and yet he grows richer. And there is one who keeps what he should give, but he ends up needing more. The man who gives much will have much, and he who helps others will be helped himself" (Proverbs 11:24–25, New Living Translation). When we generously give in this manner, we fulfill the command to love and serve others, and we bring glory to God. Speaking of love, I find it most profound that the Lord taught us, "just as I have loved you, you also are to love one another" (John 13:34).

God will indeed hold us accountable for what we do know yet casually dismiss. As we learn to embrace that nothing we have is ours, it will become easier and easier to dispose of anything we steward as God so pleases. After all, it was never ours. As we individually and collectively kingdom-shrink, our generosity can really show the world that we don't need the empty things of this world because Jesus is more than enough—He is without question all that we could ever need.

CHAPTER 20

··

LIFE IS BUT A VAPOR

Each of our lives is positioned like a bow, drawn across the strings of a cosmic violin, producing vibrations that resound for all eternity. The slightest action of the bow produces a sound, a sound that is never lost. What I do today has tremendous bearing on eternity. Indeed, it is the stuff of which eternity is made. The everyday choices I make regarding money and possessions are of eternal consequence.

—Randy Alcorn

YOUR TIME ON EARTH IS LIKE AN AIRPORT LAYOVER

To maximize what we've learned about biblical stewardship, we must understand its urgency in light of the brevity of our lives. Otherwise, we will fail to wisely invest not just the resources but also the time God has entrusted to us. Think about this reality: this second—this very moment—will become *the place* where your past intersects your future . . . forever. It is imperative that we live on purpose each and every day. This chapter provides practical ideas for you to intentionally redeem the time as you resolve to live backward and make this vapor of life count for God's glory.

Picture the following: beautiful blue skies, gently swaying palm trees, sun-drenched beaches, crystal-clear water, breathtaking panoramic views, and you in a comfortable hammock with your favorite beverage. These elements conjure up an inviting tropical paradise with all the makings of a perfect getaway.

Now imagine that you're on a layover en route to this exotic location. During the layover you might purchase a snack or magazine, read a book, take a nap, or watch the overhead television. However, you wouldn't settle into a chair and begin turning over in your mind how you can transform the airport into your destination. That would be ludicrous. Rather, you'd be keenly aware that the airport stay is only temporary and not your final destination. At all times, you'd be cognizant about where you're headed. Instead of harboring a desire to stay in the airport, you'd be in a constant state of readiness to depart: you'd be extremely alert, staying near the gate, actively checking monitors, and straining to hear PA announcements about any potential changes. Most likely, you'd be so excited about your destination that you'd scarcely be able to sit down long enough to read a book or take a nap.

We may liken the time spent on this brief layover to our relatively brief stay on the earth. We are en route to an unparalleled place called Heaven: "But we are citizens of heaven, where the Lord Jesus Christ lives. And we are eagerly waiting for him to return as our Savior" (Philippians 3:20, New Living Translation). As its citizens, we should always be aware that we're here on this earth only temporarily. Our focus, therefore, should always be drawn to *where we are going*, not to *where we currently are*. Allowing this truth to shape our thinking and our lives enables us to maximize the gift of hindsight.

UNPARALLELED EXCITEMENT

The Bible teaches with great clarity that each and every person will live forever. The only question is a matter of where: in Heaven or in Hell. Every person alive is currently on a spiritual layover. One hundred percent of people are destined to stop breathing someday. Hebrews 9:27 states, "It is appointed for man to die once, and after that comes judgment." Followers of Christ are assured that at the moment our heart stops beating, our spirits and souls will be with God in the eternal paradise He has prepared for us. I must emphasize that Heaven will be the final destination of *only those* who have trusted Christ as Savior. Contrary to what is spoken at most funerals I've attended, people don't die and automatically go to Heaven just because others think (or they themselves thought) that they had led a good and productive life. As we've already mentioned, no one can enter Heaven based on his or her merit (see Romans 3:12).

It's been said that we were made for one place and for one person. Heaven is that place, and Jesus is that person! He's promised that He's prepared a home for us whose beauty and grandeur we can't possibly begin to imagine. The excitement that we'd have for the tropical paradise should pale in comparison to the joyful expectation we should have for our glorious heavenly home. Pick the most beautiful destination on earth, and it would be but a faint echo of the splendor of our eternal home—in God's presence where there will be no tears, no pain, no sorrow, no sickness, and no heartache. Yet the reality is that many followers of Christ are so enamored with the glamorous things of this life that they do not long for Heaven. What does it say to the world when disciples aren't looking forward to being home with their Savior and King? By this question, I'm certainly not suggesting that we should wish or pray to die; I'm simply saying that we should be eager and ready to go Home whenever God calls us to.

We are merely passing through this world. James 4:14 says, "What is your life? You are a mist that appears for a little time and then vanishes." Embracing that our lives are as a vapor, we must be as vigilant as we'd be while awaiting a connecting flight. We should continuously be in a state of readiness by reading and studying God's Word, wearing the full armor of God (see Acts 17:11; Ephesians 6:10–17), walking out Christlikeness, and actively seeking to advance God's kingdom on earth. Instead of settling down and becoming totally comfortable with the world's plan and dictates for our lives, we must be faithful stewards of the time God has entrusted us, wisely investing it and doing the work God has predestined each of us to do (see Ephesians 5:15–17). We must also view everything in the light of God's eternal perspective, not in the dimness of the world's system or our finite minds.

DRESS REHEARSAL

I've heard it said, "Life is a dress rehearsal." If this means that this life is preparation for what comes after, then there's much wisdom in this maxim. However, it would be false and very misleading if we interpreted this saying to mean that we get a second chance to do an actual (or another) performance here on earth. According to the Bible, we get only one shot at this temporal life. That's it—this life is our one and only opportunity to impinge on all eternity. There's absolutely no second chance after we take our final breath. There's no purgatory, no reincarnation, or anything else of the sort. If this were not true—if we were allowed another chance to "do it again" in "another performance"—then there's no incentive for us to maximize our time and live according to God's Word in the here and now. Living backward would be meaningless.

Because of its finality, it might be even better to think of this life as both the dress rehearsal and the actual performance all wrapped up into one. Each of us is on center stage with a specific part to play, and our "performance" is incredibly brief—far briefer than we tend to think. Picture the steam coming from a kettle of boiling water. It rises into the air, but in a matter of seconds you no longer see it: this is the sheer brevity of our lives. Yet how many of us engage life as though our presence on the grand stage of life is but a passing mist?

A line from a very popular movie, *The Curious Case of Benjamin Button*, says, "It's never too late to be who you want to be." On the contrary, there will come a time when it certainly will be too late to become who you want to be. While this quote aims to give hope, it is an example of subtle, worldly thinking that unobtrusively misleads, undermining our resolve to live intentionally each and every day. Indeed, it is difficult to live backward when we have the mind-set that we have time to later become who we want to be. As I mentioned in Chapter 1 of this book, this forward perspective of time is to our peril—each day that we accrue also means that we have one less day to create significance in our lives. It's imperative to wisely value and make the most of the time entrusted to us.

Here's another way to consider the urgency of redeeming your time. Imagine that you moved as an adult to a foreign country and had to live there for a few years, after which you would return to your native country and live for eternity. In accordance with this pre-established arrangement, the only material possessions that you could bring back with you to your native land is what you sent back while you were living in the foreign country. While in the foreign country, you have the freedom to use your time, skills, and abilities to work and be equitably compensated. Any money that you earn can be invested in only one of two ways: you can keep what is necessary to meet your short-term needs and send the remainder back to a bank in your native country, or you can spend all the money that you've earned to maintain a very nice lifestyle, sending little or no money back to your native country. You can't take any money that you've earned with you when you return to your native land—it must be sent ahead. And you can't take any possessions with you at all.

What would you do? Would you send as much of the money that you've earned to your native country, keeping only what you needed to live comfortably? Or would you, having met your living expenses, spend the remaining money on the purchase of all sorts of wonderful amenities in the foreign country?

Heaven is our native country where we'll eventually exist for all eternity. Earth is the foreign country where we temporarily reside. When we consider that this present world is temporary and the life hereafter is forever, we should be strongly motivated to live in such a way so as to store up treasures in Heaven. As followers of Christ, not living for the things of this transient world *and* storing up treasures above is equivalent to wisely saving money in the foreign country (that could have been frivolously spent on material goods) and sending it to our native country.

And just as amassing treasures in the foreign country in favor of saving money and sending it to one's native country would be sheer folly, so is spending hard-earned money to buy unnecessary goods on earth that are fleeting. Yet this is exactly what we do when we fail to live with an eternal perspective of money and possessions. Instead of storing treasures above, we end up erroneously storing them here on earth. Indeed, the time will come when we, as disciples of Christ, will go to our native country, either after death or upon Christ's return. At that moment, our earthly treasures—trinkets actually—will become utterly useless; we won't be able to take any money or material possessions with us. The "stuff" that awaits us in Heaven will be what we have sent on ahead.

NOT MAKING A CHOICE IS A CHOICE

So what keeps the money God has entrusted to us more tied to this world rather than invested in His kingdom where it can become treasures, which are ours forever? The answer is fairly simple: unless we adopt the right attitude toward money and intentionally choose to store treasures above, by default we will end up storing treasures in the earth.

This is a good place to revisit the account in Matthew 6:19–24, where Jesus commands us to store treasures above. The idea of money being utilized as a tool to serve one of two purposes is its central theme. Twice in this teaching, two choices are presented: store treasures in Heaven or store them on earth; serve money or serve God. In both cases, we must select one; there is no third option. However, just as God's command that we worship nothing else besides Him is also fundamentally for our benefit, so is this teaching—God intends it for our future personal gain. Notice that Jesus doesn't say we should not store up treasures. As a matter of fact, He commands us to! We just aren't supposed to stockpile these treasures on earth.

We overlook the astounding promise of eternal rewards in this commandment. We naturally want to know how we stand to benefit from doing or not doing something before we are motivated into action—what's in it for me? The great news is that we can actually view God's command to store up eternal treasures with this "what's in it for me?" mentality. Rooted in a sincere desire to ultimately please God, this attitude is actually not wrong; it's actually a God-sanctioned perspective commended by Jesus.

God uses rewards to motivate His children just like earthly parents. God actually commands us to actively pursue future or eternal rewards (see Luke 12:33, 14:14–15, 16:1–13). It's His idea, not ours. Therefore, to actively seek eternal rewards is entirely scriptural, and to not do so is to disobey God's Word. This truth contradicts many erroneous teachings in Christianity today that suggest that it is selfish or unscriptural to pursue personal gain with regard to eternal rewards. Such teachings simply don't align with Scripture. Instead, they help further Satan's agenda to keep God's people deceived about matters of grave eternal importance.

Since Jesus commands us to store up treasures in Heaven, let's obediently do just that. Let's get excited about the prospects of storing up our treasures there and not here. After all, the sooner we start investing in eternity, the more treasures we'll have awaiting us there. But to do so, we must take to heart that we cannot continue living as if the choices we make in this temporal life won't have eternal consequences. Three things distract us from making good choices: misconceptions, wrong assumptions, and false teachings. We must discover and overcome these if we are to cultivate an eternal mind-set.

THE FINAL TEST

Many followers either misunderstand or only give mental assent to the fact that all believers will be judged for what they have done in the body, whether good or bad. Many completely overlook that the result of this judgment will be the gain or loss of eternal rewards (see Romans 14:10–12; 1 Corinthians 3:12–15, 5:9–10). This means that, though Christians are forgiven of their sins and will go to Heaven, they can still lose or forfeit rewards. The Bible tells us that each and every one of our works will be tested by fire on that great day. Only the works that were built on the foundation of Christ will last. Everything else will be burned and destroyed, and the believer will "suffer loss" (see 1 Corinthians 3:12–15). As C. T. Studd wrote, "Only one life t'will soon be past; only what's done for Christ will last." We simply don't realize just how many eternal rewards we are daily forfeiting because of the choices we both make and fail to make.

Another teaching relating to eternal rewards that many misunderstand is the parable of the sheep and the goats in Matthew 25:31–46. According to this account, when the Son of Man comes in His glory, He will separate people as a shepherd separates the sheep from the goats. The sheep will be those who provided for the needs of the hungry, thirsty, naked, imprisoned, and sick. The goats will be those who failed to demonstrate compassion to those in need. The sheep will be invited to receive their inheritance in Jesus's eternal kingdom, while the goats will be told, "Depart from me, you cursed, into the eternal fire prepared for the devil and his angels" (Matthew 41). What does this selection process of eternal magnitude say to us if we're not seeking to help minimize the inequities that abound? We can't simply dismiss Jesus's teaching that helping others in this life is an inherent characteristic displayed by His sheep. Compassion toward the needs of the poor and downtrodden goes hand in hand with being a true follower of Christ (see James 1:27). It's actually an identifying attribute of those who are truly righteous.

I didn't comprehend this spiritual truth for a very long time after I accepted Christ as my Lord. Although many of us engage life uninformed of this reality, it is not optional. Scripture mandates that a disciple actively and consistently demonstrate compassion toward the needy as Jesus did when He was on the earth.

Furthermore, we see from both the Old and New Testaments that God passionately desires to alleviate the suffering of those who are poor and in need (see Leviticus 19:9–10; Deuteronomy 15:10–11; Isaiah 58:7; Luke 14:12 –14; James 2:14–16). Not surprisingly, helping to relieve suffering in the world is one of the key ways that God has ordained for us to store up treasures. Jesus has also reassured us that each and every true act of compassion and kindness done "for the least of these" will someday be rewarded (Matthew 25:40).

Indeed, God will reward us for each and every thing we do by His inspiration to advance His kingdom on earth, even if it goes unnoticed by man. So in helping others by using that which God has entrusted to us, not only can we experience joy, but we can also be assured that we are wisely investing in our eternal portfolio. Living backward is to live with the understanding that not only is faith without works dead (see James 2:26), but that faith without works will likely result in little or no treasures in Heaven.

Another potential hurdle we face in this area of storing up treasures is that it's very easy to stop at the first part of Jesus's command in Matthew 6:19, which teaches us to not store treasures on earth. As in the above allegory, it's not enough to wisely spend money on genuine needs in the foreign country while forgoing the purchase of unnecessary "stuff," simply to save the remainder. This is only half of good stewardship. I have personally been guilty of doing just that. I became resolute in my desire to not accumulate stuff on earth but at times lost sight of the other half of the command to actually send treasures ahead. While I'm still not where I desire to be in this area, God is helping me to make progress.

Therefore, we must fulfill both parts of Jesus's command if we are to truly store up treasures in Heaven. We must recognize that not storing up treasures on earth is not an end in itself; rather, it is a temporal means to an eternal end. At the point of our death, the opportunity to store up eternal treasures will abruptly come to an end.

SENDING TREASURES AHEAD

Since life is so fleeting, and, like me, many of us have been slow to store up treasures, the remainder of this chapter is devoted to the nuts and bolts of storing up eternal rewards. It bears repeating that unless we deliberately heed Jesus's words to store treasures above and not serve money, we will by default serve money and store treasures on earth.

We've seen that how we use money clearly reveals where our heart is (see Matthew 6:21). So, ultimately, where we choose to invest or store our treasures is based on where we consider to be our home. This earth is not our home; Heaven is. Luke 12:33 suggests that eternal rewards are inexhaustible, eternal, incorruptible, and imperishable! By investing in eternal treasures, we can use resources—that could otherwise be spent on mere earthly treasures—to create an eternal investment portfolio that continues to pay dividends evermore.

We can view storing treasures in terms of two distinct financial vehicles: a temporal vehicle, which will ultimately be worthless when Christ returns or calls us home, and an eternal vehicle, which will have eternal value and worth. But unlike the real world, there's no such thing as a hybrid financial plan where we can capitalize on the best of two or more vehicles combined. We must choose the eternal vehicle if we intend to live backward.

Thankfully, God is not only our CEO; He is also our Chief Investment Officer (CIO). We are simply His financial managers, called to cooperate with Him in running His (not our) financial affairs. Our CIO is not only wise but also very kind and caring. He knows that for the sake of *our own self-interests*, it is best to aggressively invest in His everlasting kingdom, not in the kingdom of this passing world.

Therefore, He's given us Jesus, the premier Chief Financial Advisor (CFA) the world has ever known, to help us optimize our investment portfolio. From everlasting to everlasting, Jesus is all-wise and all-knowing. Absolutely nothing in all creation is hidden from Him, "but all are naked and exposed to the eyes of him to whom we must give account" (Hebrews 4:13). He is fully aware of each and every detail of our individual moment-by-moment gains and losses.

Not only that, He also knows of the great future economic doomsday, ushered in by His unannounced return at the end of the world. As His followers, we are privy to divine insider information: when He returns (if we haven't been called home prior), any money in our temporal financial vehicles will become utterly worthless.

We can either die and leave worldly trinkets here, to our eternal regret, or send treasures on ahead, to our eternal joy. Have you heard the saying, "You never see a hearse pulling a U-Haul"? This is why our CFA, Jesus, strongly advises us to wisely trade the stocks and bonds of temporal money and possessions for eternal stocks that we can never lose. People invested in the world's stock market are advised to think long term—twenty, thirty, forty years ahead. Our CFA advises us to think long term as well, beyond what our minds can even conceive:

millions upon billions of years into endless eternity. If you're a smart investor and have this long-term investment mentality, it is foolish not to choose the investment vehicle that pays and will continue to pay dividends forever.

No doubt, the kingdom of Heaven is absolutely the wisest and safest place for us to invest the money entrusted to us by God. Stocks pay returns of roughly 10 percent over the long term, but in Matthew 19:29, Jesus promises a *hundredfold* return on our investment! Clearly, the greatest return on any other earthly investment vehicle is child's play compared to God's eternal investment plan. If this scriptural reality does not appeal to our own self-interests, what should? What will? The prospect of eternal rewards is fitting motivation for structuring our investment portfolios according to Jesus's sound investment teachings.

Of course, we can also earn rewards for our good works. Ephesians 2:10 states, "For we are his workmanship, created in Christ Jesus for good works, which God prepared beforehand, that we should walk in them." All of these good works are intended to advance the kingdom of God. They involve using the gifts, time, money, resources, and possessions God has entrusted us to be channels of His grace to help others. Scripture also teaches that "whatever good anyone does, this he will receive back from the Lord" (Ephesians 6:8). God has promised to reward us for every single thing we do out of the desire to obey and please Him: every thoughtful gesture, every charitable donation, every act of service, every extended hand of help, and every word of encouragement.

THE MOST IMPORTANT DECISION

Remember, the Bible teaches that when we die we will end up spending eternity in one of two places: either in Heaven, where we will experience eternal life in the glorious presence of God, or in Hell, where we will be completely and forever separated from God in eternal condemnation.

The Bible graphically describes Hell as the lake of fire, a horrible place of damnation and darkness where the fire never goes out and where there will be perpetual weeping and gnashing of teeth (see Matthew 8:12, 10:28, 13:40–42, 22:13, 25:30; Mark 9:43–44; 2 Thessalonians 1:9). No semblance of God's grace will be there. While on earth "he [God]makes his sun rise on the evil and on the good, and sends rain on the just and on the unjust" (Matthew 5:45) and "The Lord is good to all, and his mercy is over all that he has made" (Psalm 145:9). Both verses teach that every single person living on earth continually experiences a certain measure of God's goodness, sometimes referred to as "common grace." Whether it is a tranquil night's sleep, having a secure job, recovery from an illness, the joy children and grandchildren bring, friendships, cherished memories, or protection, each of us experiences God's grace in our lives daily. In Hell, these realities will no longer be the case—we cannot even begin to conceive what it will be like there.

Contrary to many false assumptions about Heaven, it will not be a place where everyone enjoys the same status and privileges. Neither will we be accorded the same commendation with regards to treasures and responsibilities. Likewise, the Bible teaches that there will be varying degrees of punishment for those eternally separated from God in Hell. For example, Luke 12:47–48 teaches that the servant who knows his master's will but does not do it will receive more blows (see also Matthew 11:20–24; Luke 20:46–47; Romans 2:3–5). Wherever we are bound, since God is perfectly just, He will judge us with perfect fairness and knowledge. Whatever we receive in either place will be determined by what we have both known and sown in this life. So though our character will not determine where we spend eternity, it will nonetheless condition the quality of our eternal well-being. This eternal status is what we should be unwaveringly pursuing, not the fleeting status found in the material goods and pleasures of this world.

Our payday in Heaven will be based on the godly quality of our lives here on earth, how many treasures we sent ahead, and how much our lives mattered for God and His kingdom. More will be ours to claim if we choose to live on earth with a reverse perspective of time. Our individual experiences in Heaven will vary greatly depending on the quality and quantity of rewards that we receive. All of God's children will indeed be there, but many distinctions will exist based on whether we have acted in the capacity of a good steward, diligently serving His master with what was entrusted to him, or as if an owner of the master's rightful property, usurping the master's ownership by doing whatever we pleased.

TURNED TABLES

There's a biblical teaching referred to as the Great Reversal: in Heaven many will have positions that will be the opposite of what they had on earth. For example, the person of modest means who lived generously, obediently, and sacrificially all his life will have more eternal rewards than the rich person who merely lived for himself and did very little to help others. This reversal will also occur regarding who is considered great in Heaven. Those whom the world considers remarkable may not be esteemed in Heaven; those who are humble and serve others on the earth will assuredly be the greatest in God's kingdom (see Mark 9:35, 10:43). However, it's very important to point out that, despite there being varying degrees of rewards, the joy of each person in Heaven will be full and complete for all eternity—but Scripture suggests that we will likely experience varying degrees of that joy.

We also would do well to remember Jesus's words: "One who is faithful in a very little is also faithful in much, and one who is dishonest in a very little is also dishonest in much" (Luke 16:10). What we do with a little time, or a little money, says a lot about the kind of steward we truly are; Jesus warned, "If then you have not been faithful in the unrighteous wealth, who will entrust to you the true riches?" (Luke 16:11). These true riches are ones of eternal value; that which we may think of as little is actually significant in the eyes of God. The rewards and positions we receive in His eternal kingdom will be based on how we've handled the littlest of things here on the earth. As John Wesley stated, we must come to "value all things by the price they shall gain in eternity."[49]

ANYONE CAN INDEED BE GREAT

I conclude this book with exciting news. The Bible does not teach that we need to have boatloads of money in order to store up treasures. Instead, "If anyone would be first, he must be last of all and servant of all" (Mark 9:35). The same teaching is repeated in Mark 10:43–45: "But whoever would be great among you must be your servant, and whoever would be first among you must be slave of all. For even the Son of Man came not to be served but to serve, and to give his life as a ransom for many." We should always reverentially heed God's words, but when God repeats Himself, how much more should we pay close attention to that teaching? Being a servant to all now is not optional for us if we want to be great in God's eyes in eternity. Jesus poignantly modeled this attribute for us when he humbly reversed roles and washed the feet of His disciples. We're called to do no less.

The Bible undeniably teaches that true humility is true greatness. So the great news for you and me is that any one of us can be great— very great—because any one of us can serve. With specific regard to storing up treasures, it also means that because any one of us can serve others, especially those in need, we all can store up an abundance of eternal treasures in obedience to God and as led by His Spirit.

A glorious, eternal future awaits you and me! How exciting that every promise of eternal reward in God's Word is brimming with the fact that God delights in commending us for our obedience. Shouldn't we be equally motivated about receiving these rewards? C. S. Lewis

---

49. Cited in Randy Alcorn, *Money, Possessions, and Eternity* (Wheaton: Tyndale House Publishers, Inc., 2003), 94.

summed up God's lavish blessing for those who follow Him and delight in Him: "Indeed, if we consider the unblushing promises of reward promised in the Gospels, it would seem that our Lord finds our desires not too strong, but too weak."[50] Today, how would He find your desire?

I pray we become increasingly motivated to possess all that God has for us through Christ our Lord. Ultimately, storing our treasures above honors and pleases God. In 1 Peter 5:6, we are admonished: "Humble yourselves, therefore, under the mighty hand of God so that at the proper time he may exalt you." Indeed, God will honor in Heaven those who have honored Him on the earth.

In the meantime, He has set us apart to live for Him here, earnestly and unashamedly pursuing our core destiny in Christ. This is what matters most! So no matter if you attain a stellar GPA, are an amazingly gifted athlete, live in the most luxurious of homes, boast a litany of credentials, ascend to the top of the corporate ladder, achieve the zenith of your profession, marry the person of your dreams, raise smart and successful children, have all the money you could ever desire, or attain worldly fame, nothing you can ever do will truly matter or retain eternal significance outside of conforming your life to Christ.

Scripture gives this warning, and it is the conclusion of the matter: "Unless the Lord builds the house, those who build it labor in vain" (Psalm 127:1).

If you don't live backward *in the now*, you will forfeit significance where it eternally matters—*in Heaven*. Eternity is a very, very, very long time to live with the regret of how you *could have or should have* lived this life.

Starting right this moment, resolve to let your life count for that which nothing else is greater or higher—God's glory. Seize the gift of future-oriented hindsight so that when you stand before your Creator, you'll experience the eternal joy and satisfaction of having built a truly significant life!

Remember . . . I'm cheering you on!

....

50. C. S. Lewis, *The Weight of Glory* (New York: HarperCollins, 1980), 26.

EPILOGUE

I've heard it said, "A belief is what you hold; a conviction is what holds you." At some point, the convictions we hold in our hearts, coupled with all that God has graciously poured into us, must rouse us into action. They must find practical expression in our hands and feet if we are to truly make a difference for Christ in the world. Inevitably, the path of following Jesus leads us straight into a broken and hurting world, for our Lord and King has issued this decree, "Give as freely you have received" (Matthew 10:8, New Living Translation). God desires to fill us up so that we may go into a needy world and fill up others with the love and grace that He has shown us. Therefore, those things that grieve the heart of the living God must grieve ours till it moves our hands and feet into action; they must break our hearts till the river of our compassion flows into the dry and barren valleys, carrying the Good News to the lost and meeting in practical ways the needs of the thirsty, hungry, hopeless, brokenhearted, and downtrodden.

Carrying out this boldness and passion for Christ angers the enemy of our souls. Even though Satan is ever and always subject to God, God has, nevertheless, temporarily given Him power in the earth (see Galatians 1:4; 2 Corinthians 4:4). He is relentless in his efforts and attempts to abort God's plan in our lives, as well as God's purposes in the world. In 2 Chronicles 20:15, it states, "The battle is not ours but God's"—we know that ultimately we are triumphant because of the blood of Christ. However, Scripture also teaches that we must be vigilant against the devil (see Ephesians 6:12). Although a full discussion of spiritual warfare went beyond the scope of this book, I want you to always bear in mind that we are in a daily battle with Satan. *The Art of War,* written roughly two thousand years ago, is an ancient Chinese military treatise attributed to Sun Tzu, a high-ranking military general, strategist, and technician. Considered the most definitive work on military strategy and tactics of its time, it has influenced (and continues to influence) both eastern and western military thinking and strategy. I'd like to leave you with a quote from *The Art of War* that saliently captures the importance of knowing well the tactics and schemes of our mortal enemy:

> If you know the enemy and know yourself, you need not fear the result of a hundred battles. If you know yourself but not the enemy, for every victory gained you will also suffer a defeat. If you know neither the enemy nor yourself, you will succumb in every battle.

God's people "are a chosen race, a royal priesthood, a holy nation, a people for his own possession, that [we] may proclaim the excellencies of him who called [us] out of darkness into his marvelous light" (1 Peter 2:9). My prayer is that you will take what you've learned from this book and go forward in leading a joy-filled, victorious, and Christ-exalting life, to the honor and glory of our Father in Heaven. Of this, He is infinitely worthy, forever and ever!

ACKNOWLEDGMENTS

First and foremost, to the triune God: God my Father, Jesus my Savior, and my Helper, the sweet Holy Spirit—if I had a thousand tongues I still couldn't thank you enough. My deepest passion is to ever love you, please you, and delight your heart. It is only by your sheer grace that this book came to be.

To my tremendous parents, E. J. Llewellyn Cooper, Sr., and Isabel Simpson Cooper: Although you both have made your spiritual transitions, I am overjoyed that God chose you for my parents. Words can never fully capture how very much I adore you, nor can they express my appreciation for the innumerable sacrifices you both made for our family. Who I am today is in large part the result of the firm yet loving and nurturing environment in which you raised my siblings and me. Thank you immensely Daddy and Mommie, for instilling in me godly values and for helping to lay the groundwork for God to later move mightily in my life. I love and miss you beyond words.

This book has been an incredible labor of love. It exists in large part because of what many others before me have written and shared. I'm most thankful for spiritual giants of the past from whom I've gleaned so much knowledge and wisdom.

I would be remiss if I did not thank my four favorite current authors. To Randy Alcorn, Jerry Bridges, Elisabeth Elliott, and John Piper: Although fulfilling, writing to truly help others learn and grow is difficult and laborious. Thank you ever so much for being an instrument of God and obediently answering His call on your lives. Your writings have been instrumental in helping to shape my understanding of God and His desires for me. My love and passion for our God and King has been greatly stirred by your ardent love and passion.

To Stephanie Smith of Zondervan Publishing: Thank you for your time and for believing in the message of *Living Backward*. This was not the book's original title. So I owe you a huge vote of thanks for graciously challenging me to come up with a more unique title as well as a salient angle for the manuscript.

To Stan Gundry of Zondervan Publishing: You are an incredibly kind man! Your words of affirmation and demonstrated belief in me went a long way toward building my confidence as a first-time non-fiction author. Thanks so very much for helping me to get my foot in the door and for your wise counsel and feedback. I took your advice to keep plugging forward until the book was published.

To my developmental editor, Melissa Wuske: From our very first phone call, I knew you were just the right editor for this book. And from there on you continued to solidify my trust in your excellent editorial skills. Your thoughtful questions, insightful comments, and suggestions for improvement were invaluable. Like clay in the hands of an expert potter, you helped mold and shape the contents of this book, refining the manuscript and taking it to the next level. Throughout it all you were extremely kind, professional, highly responsive, and a pleasure to work with. Thanks for believing in the merit of this book and for your kind words of encouragement. You have played a key role in preparing *Living Backward* for its introduction to the literary marketplace for which I'm most grateful.

To the stellar Girl Friday Productions team: It has been such a pleasure working with you all to produce *Living Backward*. Christina

Henry de Tessan, you were the first person I spoke with, and it was truly a delightful conversation. I'll always remember the warmth and professionalism you exuded. Thank you for placing me in the capable and thorough hands of Meghan Harvey who was in a word, amazing—from beginning to end. Meghan, I so appreciate the kind and gracious manner that you shepherded me through the entire process. You're the best! To my wonderful copyeditor, Michelle Hope Andersen, I'm grateful for your thoughtful comments and suggestions for improvement. They helped to further refine the manuscript. Paul Barrett, I appreciate your creativity, your responsiveness, and your design work for the book's cover and interior—very nice work! Thank you, Carrie Wicks, for efficiently proofreading the manuscript. To the lovely Andrea Dunlop, thanks so much for your expertise and kind input along the way. To Stephanie Billings, Ingrid Emerick, and everyone else at GFP who worked behind the scenes or had a hand in making *Living Backward* a reality: thank you. Your collective efforts made me feel valued and well cared for.

To each and every one—family, friend, or acquaintance—who prayed for me or offered encouragement along the way: thank you so much.

To my beloved siblings and their families (including my wonderful nieces and nephews): Emma Holder (now deceased), Patience and Terry Saines, Ethelbert and Bendu Cooper, Joy and Emmette Burnette, Juliet and Henry Allen, Daubeny and Anita Cooper, and Isabel J. Cooper: Thank you for your love, prayers, encouragement, and support down through the years. I'm grateful for a lifetime of beautiful memories, and I love each of you very much.

To Julia Yates: While chatting several years ago, you enthusiastically suggested that I should write a book. Although I already knew that I wanted to write a book someday, something about your warm, spirited remark left an impression on me. Thanks so much for encouraging me to pursue this call of God on my life.

To Christie Clark: thank you for your willingness to read some of the manuscript and for providing helpful comments.

To Diane Lowery: Thank you for being willing to review and edit part of the manuscript. I appreciate your editorial help and comments.

To my lovely niece, Jessica Allen Bernthal: You are a talented writer. Thank you for taking the time to give a quick look over the draft of my manuscript and for your kind and encouraging words. Most of all, thank you for boldly pointing out to your aunt the need for her to reinvent her writing style so as to make it more suitable for today's readers. It was truly a nugget of wisdom. I love you very much.

To my sweet niece, Tanya Cooper Mathieu: Thank you for your willingness to have read the manuscript. Your words of affirmation were not only humbling, but also a huge boost to my spirit. I'm so grateful to God that you were blessed in the process. I love you very much.

To my brother-in-love, Dr. Henry Lee Allen: Heartfelt thanks for believing in me and this book. You opened a door for me that I otherwise wouldn't have been able to walk through. I love and appreciate you.

To my sweet sister, Juliet Cooper Allen: I'm so grateful that God saw fit to give me such a smart, loving, creative, and gifted sister. Thank you for reading some of the earlier manuscript and for your helpful comments and ideas as I worked to refine it. Your belief in the book's message encouraged me. Also, thank you so much for taking me to weekly Bible studies as an adolescent. Seeds planted during those times are bearing fruit today. I love and treasure you!

To my darling sister, Isabel J. Cooper: I'm glad to have grown up doing everything with you, and I'm so grateful to God for the special bond that we share. Thank you for believing in *Living Backward*, giving me good feedback, and cheering me on. Your constant love, kindness, and ongoing support mean the world to me. I love and treasure you!

To Cindy Ratzlaff: You were a godsend to me. Thank you from the bottom of my heart for believing in me as an author as well as the message of *Living Backward.* I'm very grateful for your time, your kindness, and the fantastic people with whom you've connected me.

To Lisa McKenzie: You are absolutely delightful! I admire your passion for what you do and feel so blessed and privileged to be working with you. Every time you speak, I hang on to your every word and marvel at the breadth of your knowledge and expertise. Thank you so very much for your creative input. I'll always be deeply grateful to you for helping me to crystallize the book's subtitle. We make a great team! *Merci beaucoup*: encore!

To Jim Edwards: thank you very much for your willingness to read the entire manuscript and provide helpful feedback.

To my wonderful friends and sisters in Christ, Lauren Alexander, Traci Davis, Cate McKenzie, and Karen Snuffer: Thanks so much for taking time out of your busy schedules to serve as beta readers for the final draft of this book. I greatly appreciate your kindness and willingness to assist me in this tangible way. Each of you provided great input by helping to identify statements that needed more clarification or pointing out things that helped round out what I endeavored to convey. This book is better because of your collective comments and suggestions. Thanks so much for all the kind and encouraging words interspersed throughout your feedback. I love each of you very much and greatly appreciate you.

To my dear friend and sister in Christ, Christie Pride: Amid a most demanding schedule, you kindly agreed to be a beta reader. But you went above and beyond beta reading—employing your wonderful writing skills, you became an unofficial editor of sorts, evidenced by the keen insights and comments that you provided. I'm so very grateful for your help in the preliminary refining of the book's contents. It went to my editor in much better shape than it otherwise would have been. Thank you for your love, ongoing prayers, and support. I value our friendship, and I love and appreciate you very much.

To Jillian Alexander, "my daughter from another mother": You deserve a medal of perseverance for poring through the very first draft of this book. How very rough a manuscript it was at the time! Yet you graciously gave of your time and energies to edit it and give me helpful feedback. I now know more than ever just how much of a labor of love it was. And I'll never forget your kindness! I thank God for the beautiful ways that you reflect His image, and I love you very much.

To my dear friend and sister in Christ, Pamela Taylor: You were the first person to read the book's introduction and provide me feedback. Your kind words of affirmation inspired and spurred me on. You believed in the message of *Living Backward* right from the start. I'll never forget our lunches at Panera's. Thank you for your love, constant prayers, encouragement, and support. And thank you for believing in me. Your friendship is a beautiful gift from God, and I love you very much.

To Cate McKenzie: Besides being a beta reader, thank you so much for being in my corner and always cheering me on. You were instrumental in bringing about a critical shift in my perspective that enabled me to write more effectively for the readers of this book. For this I thank you from the bottom of my heart. Big thanks also for time and again reminding me that this book "matters for God." Hearing you affirm my zeal to *matter for God* always gave me a huge boost—both spiritually and physically! You've been simply wonderful!

To my longtime friend and sister in Christ, Etmonia Benjamin: You believed in the relevance and message of this book from the very first moment that I shared it with you. Ever since that time, you've been one of my biggest fans, enthusiastically cheering me on. Your love, faithfulness, commitment to keep me covered in your prayers, words of encouragement, and support throughout this writing project have all carved an even bigger space in my heart for you. Thank you for wholeheartedly believing in me. You are a special gift from God. I love you very much and cherish our friendship.

To Paris Green, my wonderful brother in Christ: Thank you so much for being a beta reader. It didn't stop there, though. You were truly a godsend while I wrote this book! You had a knack for reaching out to me at just the right time—when I most needed a boost of encouragement. Indeed, your calls and texts were like a drink of ice-cold water on a sweltering day; your God-exalting prayers refreshed and energized me. Thanks for always pointing me to Scripture. I deeply appreciate all the words of hope and inspiration that you've shared along the way. And from the bottom of my heart I'm grateful for your heartfelt prayers, friendship, encouragement, and support.

To my dear brother, Bert: You are simply amazing! At twelve, God used you to literally save my life. Since that time, you've continued to bless me in innumerable ways. Dedication to family and generosity are hallmarks of your life. From the depths of my heart, thank you for believing in me and this book. Because of the countless and pivotal ways that you've blessed and enriched my life, my gratitude forever knows no bounds. I love you very much!

To Chayil, Jordan, and Jared: I'm grateful for your continual inter-est in the "book project" and for celebrating high points with me. Thanks so much for never complaining about your mother being glued to the computer while writing this book. Instead, you were most patient, understanding, and helpful, as you truly got the seriousness and importance of what I had undertaken. I always tried to give you my undivided attention when you needed me. For those times that I failed, please forgive me. I will do all that I can to make up for the times that the book took me away from being with you. Thanks for loving me so sweetly. Your spontaneous hugs and shoulder rubs, as well as your concern for me to get more sleep, meant more to me than you could ever know. I love each of you to Betelgeuse and back!

To the absolutely wonderful man that I get to call "my" husband: Your love for me is a priceless treasure, adding sparkle to my life in countless beautiful ways. I've had the joy of watching God transform you from the inside out into a truly remarkable husband, father, and man. Thank you, Honey, for your amazing servant's heart. You tenderly love me more and more fully each passing day as you seek to exemplify in our marriage the love that Christ has for His Bride. For this, I'm so very grateful. Since reading is not your thing, I greatly appreciate your reading a very rough draft of this manuscript. I believe God commissioned me to write this book. Yet I couldn't have done so without your prayers, steadfast support, and belief in me (as well as what was once only known as "the book project"). With godly patience, you cheerfully allowed me to spend hundreds of hours on the computer—while God birthed this book—that I otherwise would have spent with you. For these reasons and all the tireless sacrifices you made and continue to make so that I could write unencumbered by a job, I cannot possibly thank you enough. You fill my life with joy, and I love you beyond words. I simply love, love, love being the wife of Kyle Eugene McGlotten!

ABOUT THE AUTHOR

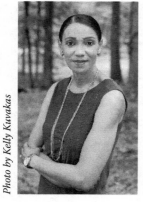

Angelique Cooper McGlotten is originally from Liberia, West Africa, where she was born and raised until a coup d'état forced her family to flee to the United States in 1980. She holds a bachelor's degree in psychology from the University of Virginia. Having woven the gift of future-oriented hindsight into her own life, she knows firsthand its power to both shape our purpose and infuse our lives with meaning. In fact, *Living Backward* is birthed from her desire to inspire others to live out God's plan for their lives and in so doing experience contentment, genuine success, and lasting significance.

Known affectionately by her family as "Triple E" (Encourager, Edifier, and Exhorter), Angelique enjoys using her gift of encouragement in a personal ministry focused on walking alongside others. She currently oversees the ministry of encouragement at the church where her husband is the founding and senior pastor, and is also the drummer for its praise and worship band. For several years, she worked alongside her husband in the Assignment, a ministry whose goal is to disciple followers of Christ, helping them discover their God-given abilities and walk in their God-given calling. Since then she has mentored (and continues to mentor) many people—adults and young adults alike through a variety of organizations. Together, she and her husband provide premarital counseling as well as lay spiritual guidance to married couples. Angelique regularly speaks at retreats, women's groups, and conferences on various topics pertaining to the Christian faith. A trained and certified facilitator, she has conducted Christian discipleship classes. She is a current board member of Care Net Pregnancy Resources, serving in the capacity of board secretary.

Angelique is the author of a book of poetry titled *The Weaver's Thread*. *Living Backward* is her first nonfiction work.

When not writing or studying, Angelique relishes time with family. She also enjoys reading, journaling, exercising, and capturing memories. She resides in northern Virginia with her husband and three children.

Angelique kindly invites you to connect with her and would love to hear your comments about this book. Please visit her author website at www.livingbackward.com.

25703063R00199

Made in the USA
Middletown, DE
07 November 2015